Relational Theory for Clinical Practice

Relational Theory for Clinical Practice offers students and practitioners a conceptual framework for thinking relationally about social work with clients within a biological, psychological, and socio-cultural framework.

Integrating relational theory with the principles of clinical practice, and demonstrating how this can be applied to social work practice, this book has been revised and updated to be suitable for students and practitioners. Using new case material to demonstrate the theory in action, this new edition of *Relational Theory for Social Work Practice: A Feminist Perspective* incorporates teaching points to aid readers in drawing out the practice principles developed in each chapter.

Keeping relationships at the center of the text, this edition includes substantially expanded chapters on assessment and intervention, and takes into account recent research on issues such as the impact of trauma and stress; neuroscience and brain research; and the necessity of practicing in a culturally sensitive way with diverse populations. It broadens the feminist focus of relational–cultural theory by extending and applying it to men also.

Designed for use on master's-level courses in practice, as well as courses on human behavior and the social environment, this concise and practical book is a valuable text for social work and counseling students.

Sharon Freedberg is an Associate Professor in the Department of Social Work, and Interim Associate Dean of the School of Health Sciences, Human Services, and Nursing at Lehman College, City University of New York, USA.

Relational Theory
for Clinical Practice

Sharon Freedberg

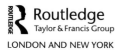

Routledge
Taylor & Francis Group

LONDON AND NEW YORK

First published 2015
by Routledge
2 Park Square, Milton Park, Abingdon, Oxon OX14 4RN

and by Routledge
711 Third Avenue, New York, NY 10017

Routledge is an imprint of the Taylor & Francis Group, an informa business

British Library Cataloguing-in-Publication Data
A catalogue record for this book is available from the British Library

Library of Congress Cataloging in Publication Data
Freedberg, Sharon, 1947-
Relational theory for clinical practice / Sharon Freedberg. -- Second edition.
pages cm
1. Social case work. I. Title.
HV43.F74 2015
361.3'201--dc23
2014030845

ISBN: 978-0-415-81450-8 (hbk)
ISBN: 978-0-415-81451-5 (pbk)
ISBN: 978-0-203-06712-3 (ebk)

Typeset in Sabon
by GreenGate Publishing Services, Tonbridge, Kent

Contents

Preface

In this second edition of *Relational Theory for Social Work Practice*, I have attempted to chart new directions in an effort to broaden and deepen the reader's understanding of the application of relational–cultural theory to clinical practice. I have included new theoretical developments and new evidence from research, re-examined the application of relational theories to clinical practice, and have added more robust case studies of diverse populations. Case studies are used to illustrate the integration of culturally sensitive relational theory with practice and present the reader with clear working guidelines.

Societies, like individuals, change over time, usually incrementally but sometimes more dramatically. Theoretical constructs are constantly fueled by new research findings, as clinical practice continues to evolve and reach new populations. As I mentioned in the first edition of this book, I was drawn to the ideas of Thomas Kuhn when Dr. Carol Meyer and Dr. Carel Germain introduced him to my doctoral class at the Columbia University School of Social Work. According to Kuhn (1970), radical changes in science do not develop through an accretion of knowledge. Rather, it is the phenomena that do not fit into current belief systems and are therefore inexplicable, that lead to new bodies of theory—what Kuhn calls paradigms. A new paradigm links rules, facts, and principles in a radically different structure to explain these anomalous phenomena.

The relational–cultural approach to practice offers a new paradigm that is especially relevant in the light of recent social changes. Emerging empirical data, research, and the changing nature of the social environment argue for the need for new theories to address new realities—changes in gender relations, changes in family structure, increased awareness of eating disorders, increased longevity and consequent social isolation, and attention to bullying as a social problem. A new paradigm which moves from the individual to social relations is timely; especially one which questions the use of male-oriented theories to explain female growth and behavior. Social work is a profession numerically dominated by women serving a largely female population. Despite the fact that feminist scholarship has proliferated, and new methodologies that are sensitive to diverse populations are evolving, the hierarchy and knowledge base still reflects a predominance of traditional male-oriented theories of development that emphasize separation/individuation rather than highlight the role that connection plays in human adaptation and development.

In its emphasis on the interactional elements of people's lives, a feminist-oriented relational approach is rooted in our professional history and harkens back to the settlement house days of Jane Addams. The method by which early social workers lived among urban settlers focused on connecting individuals to resources in the larger political cultural system through the small group and local community. In her seminal 1934 monograph *Between Client and Community*, Bertha Reynolds made explicit the importance of integrating giving help on an individual basis with community involvement and political awareness. When other psychiatrically trained workers like Reynolds were formulating individual treatment plans, the goals of which were to cure what was perceived as an illness residing in the individual, she articulated an approach to practice that addressed the need for the individual's adaptation to the community. This dual focus—on both the advancement of social justice and on individual adjustment—requires a theory that links the individual to the environment.

The emphasis on the relationship has not only been present from the very beginnings of our profession, it is also at its very heart. In her book *Relationship: The heart of helping people* (1979), Perlman writes: "It is the theme and substance of this phenomenon we call 'relationship' that is a catalyst, an enabling dynamism in the support, nurture and freeing of people's energies and motivations toward problem solving and the use of help" (p. 2). In that sense, this is a new paradigm.

In this second edition, the central premise of the book remains the same; that is, people grow and thrive best in a relational context that is mutual and reciprocal. According to the *American College Dictionary* (Barnhart, 1966), mutuality and reciprocity are synonymous; "mutuality is the distinctive idea that one party acts by way of return and response to something previously done by the other party" (p. 803). This implies that the parties involved in the interchange are actively interested in each other and are reciprocally involved in a process of mutual exchange.

In and of themselves, mutual and reciprocal relationships are not curative but are helpful in the process of change and social adaptation. Relationships characterized by mutuality and reciprocity, however, can be viewed as a protective factor in bringing about positive change and in mitigating cycles of isolation, loneliness, pain, and destruction. Protective factors have been defined in the literature as conditions, resources, coping strategies, and strengths in individuals, families, and communities that can increase the health and well-being of children and families (see Saleebey, 2006). In fact, research supports the idea that social isolation and loneliness can affect life and death. For example, in the field of gerontology, Elwert and Christakis (2008) have presented evidence that, following the death of a long-term life partner, life expectancy for the surviving person is drastically reduced.

In the field of substance abuse, Tracy et al. (2010) have researched the positive impact of relational networks on women in recovery from substance abuse. Studies of the rash of recent school shootings indicate that the perpetrators were young men who had a history of social isolation and who fit the role of social "misfits" (see Solomon, 2012).

Judith Jordan reminds us that disconnection can be viewed as a source of human suffering. I believe that as clinicians, we need to heighten our awareness of relational patterns and issues between and among individuals as well as between individuals and groups, communities, and families. This relational perspective is essential to a sound assessment and intervention plan, and we need to explore and target relational factors as focal points for change.

People have a powerful impact upon each other across the life cycle. My professional and personal experiences bear out the fact that, in working with adolescents, an absent parent often plays a greater role in the youngster's difficulties than the parent who lives with the adolescent on a daily basis. In Chapter 3, the case of Justin and Tracy illustrates how the clinician used a broader assessment of an adolescent's relational history to help a mother and her son understand the impact of the father's absence on Justin's life. While mother and son denied feelings that Justin's father held significance for him, a deeper look showed that the "forgotten" father, and his internalized image, was indeed a driving force in this adolescent boy's defiant behavior.

Early publications by the noted Stone Center psychiatrist Jean Baker Miller presented the idea (commonly referred to as "self-in-relation" theory) that the primary experience of self for women is relational. Later, self-in-relation theory came to be known as relational–cultural theory to reflect the important role that culture plays in the human experience. Contributors to relational–cultural theory include psychologists Judith V. Jordan, Janet Surrey, Maureen Walker, and social workers Julie Mencher, Wendy Rosen, and Clevonne Turner. Since the first edition, significant new work has emerged from scholars and practitioners such as Dr. Amy Banks on the neurobiology of relationships; Linda Hartling on substance abuse and prevention, shame and humiliation; and Mary Tantillo on eating disordered women and relational therapy.

The relational–cultural model provides a foundation for the case studies presented in this edition. Throughout this book the term relational theory is used interchangeably with the relational–cultural approach and the feminist relational approach. The female relational–cultural theorists and clinicians developed their approach based on the understanding that females form their sense of self in relation to others, while males have traditionally been socialized to value autonomy and independence. However, while relational–cultural theory initially relied upon scholarship based on the experiences and psychosocial development of women, it is increasingly being used to gain a better understanding of all human experience, including the importance of connection and disconnection in the lives of men and boys as well.

In this new century, gender roles are becoming increasingly fluid, and boys and men have more social permission to express their "feminine" side; that is the side that is empathic, caring, and relational. Boys and girls, and men and women, share more with regard to the need for love, social connection, empathy, acceptance, affirming relationships, and attachment than we may have been previously aware of.

As previously mentioned, throughout the history of social work, the notion of relationships has always been central to the profession's practice base; in fact, the importance of social relationships and the client worker relationship helped set it apart from other professions. Chapter 1 takes a longitudinal view of the history of social work through a relational lens. Just as the field of clinical social work espouses an ecological systems framework that views the person and situation as the interacting parts of whole, relational theories provide the link between the person and the environment. Chapter 2 provides a succinct review of relational theories including the interpersonal theory, self-psychology, ego psychology, object relations theory, intersubjective theory, and, in particular, the work on relational–cultural theory (RCT) evolving out of the Stone Center for Developmental Services and Studies at the Wellesley Centers for Women, Wellesley College. RCT builds on the work of Robert Stolorow and colleagues, and sheds new light on the interplay of the subjective experiences of both client and worker.

The main premise of RCT is the primacy of relationships in human development and bio-psycho-social functioning. This approach differs from other psychodynamic relational theories in its close attention to cultural factors, the importance placed on mutual empathy and mutual empowerment, and the role healthy connections can play in fostering healing and growth. The concept of the "relational self" places emphasis on the two-way process implicit in all relationships, including the therapeutic encounter. As is highlighted in Chapter 1, from the days of Mary Richmond, to the psychiatric-minded social workers, to Helen Harris Perlman, the social work relationship has been seen as the connecting thread that links worker and client. Chapter 3 focuses on the application of relational–cultural concepts to the client–worker relationship. New case material is used to illustrate the integration of stage trauma theory and the relational cultural approach to practice, and the way the worker used her knowledge and skills to deepen the level of trust in the client–worker relationship over time.

Empathy has been a component of social work's professional foundation for theory and practice almost since its inception. But the concept of mutual empathy is specific to RCT. Chapter 4 explores this concept and presents several cases which illustrate the reciprocal impact that client and worker have on each other. This kind of deep understanding can be very empowering for clients who might not have received this type of validation or mirroring in their early or current life—and it may help them in return to be more empathic to others.

As I have indicated, my intent in this book is to highlight the central importance of relationships between individuals and family members, between individuals and community institutions and structures, and within groups, and to show how the application of relationally oriented practice can not only facilitate the assessment process, but also direct therapeutic interventions and facilitate change. Judith Jordan reminds us that disconnection can be viewed as a source of human suffering. I believe as clinicians, we need to heighten our awareness of relational patterns and issues between and among individuals as well as between individuals and groups, communities, and families. This relational perspective is essential to a sound assessment and intervention plan, and we need to explore and target relational factors as focal points for change.

In the new edition, I discuss assessment and intervention in separate chapters which has allowed me to expand on the concepts and to include additional case material. For example, a case illustration in Chapter 5 demonstrates the assessment and planning process with a woman suffering from postpartum psychosis and the resultant consequences for her and her newborn. The clinician was able to employ relational techniques in building a support network of friends, family, and professionals to help this young woman deal with her situation. Chapter 6 presents a group of eating disordered women and shows how the integration of relational cultural theory, group theory, and knowledge of eating disorders supports change in this population.

Embedded in the relational–cultural framework for clinical practice is the idea that culture has a direct impact on the psychosocial development and functioning of the individual. Chapter 7 presents a "feminist" view on the ethics and values of the profession, with attention to the inherent tensions many women face in striking a balance between caring for oneself and giving to others. The case of Theresa illustrates just how complicated it can be for the worker to reconcile differences between her own values and the client's values, which are shaped by culture and family.

One of the most important tools a worker has is the self. I wanted to write a book in which the worker is encouraged to use that self in a creative, authentic way. The challenge of this work is not only to combine acute self-awareness with a clear differ-entiation of self, but also to be able to emotionally connect with clients in a way that is sensitive and attuned to their thoughts and feelings. It is this dance of attunement that makes the social worker, at his or her best, a flexible, skilled instrument.

Using her experience in the United Seamen's Service as a springboard, Bertha Capen Reynolds championed a vision of people working together toward solving individual and social problems. Let us not forget that social work is, first and foremost, a social profession—our history clearly speaks to this idea.

In summary, it is my hope that this review of relational–cultural theory, and the direct application to robust and richly diverse practice material, will demonstrate to the reader the importance of keeping relationships at the forefront of assessment, planning, and intervention.

Acknowledgements

I would like to acknowledge several people who have made invaluable contributions to this new edition. Without their help, this book would not have been possible.

First, I would like to thank Andrew Gottlieb and Bernice Kurchin for their editorial assistance. Their enthusiasm for this work as well as their technical help and guidance were a major source of support.

I owe a debt of gratitude to Melanie Shapiro, Andrea Raphael Paskey, and Janit Bliss for the case material they contributed to this book. These cases have enriched this work in many ways. All are skilled clinicians and consummate social workers who brought their knowledge of theory and their own relational abilities to help me illustrate the application of relational–cultural theory to clinical practice.

I also want to thank my friends; although they might not have read every chapter, their support and relational connections sustained me through this labor of love.

Special thanks to Dr. Manny Gonzalez for his belief in the importance of this book. Manny generously shared his work with me on relational–cultural theory and the Hispanic culture. Holly Fancher provided input into the section on neuroscience and was also an enthusiastic supporter of this work.

I want to thank Joseph Martinez at Lehman College for his technical assistance and Elizabeth Meister at the Wellesley Centers for Women Publications Department for her assistance in helping me obtain access to the material that I needed to complete this work.

This section would not be complete if I did not mention the members of my "knitting" group who have sustained me through different life stages. We have been meeting for over fifteen years and are still going strong.

Finally, I would like to acknowledge my daughters, Melanie and Amanda, who make me so proud of the young women they have become. I also want to welcome Skylar into the family; she elicits such joy that she gives new meaning to relationships. And thanks to Mo who gives new meaning to relational fathering. And last, but certainly not least, I would like to thank David, who painstakingly read every page of this book, helped to edit it, and offered invaluable contributions.

1 The history of social work through a relational lens

Social work has always been concerned with people and their relationships. In fact, one of the distinguishing characteristics of the social work profession is its focus on the whole person interacting with social systems in the environment—this includes relationships with family, significant others, friends, neighbors, community, work place, culture. Beginning in the last half of the nineteenth century in the pre-professional days of the Charity Organization Society (COS) movement, and continuing to the present, attention has alternated between the individual and the individual's relationships in his or her environment.

Social work has historically paid attention to relationships in its approach to helping individuals solve personal and social problems. However, the conceptualization of relational issues and their place in practice has shifted and evolved over time depending on economic, social, and political trends, and prevailing theoretical and practice approaches: such as the influences of Social Darwinism, Freud's psychoanalytic theory, advances in psychiatry and psychology, and wars and their aftermaths.

Farley et al.'s definition of social work as "an art, a science, a profession that helps people solve personal, group (especially family), and community problems and attain satisfying personal, group, and community relationships through social work practice" (2008, p. 7) is consistent with the basic assumption underlying the material presented in this chapter. Further, this chapter will take a longitudinal view of the client–worker relationship and its application to practice.

Casework before the 1920s: the attempt to "uplift"

Between the late 1800s and the early 1900s the COS movement was established as a way of helping the poor by providing an alternative to public relief. The COSs were philanthropic organizations functioning under private auspices and endowed with a moral mission of moving the poor, intemperate, and indolent toward self-sufficiency and financial independence—a goal consistent with the spirit of individualism in a capitalist society. Partly a product of the era of Social Darwinism, which fostered a belief that those who could not manage in society without help were unlikely to survive, this ideal of helping people to become self-sufficient was carried out by the societies' "friendly visitors" (Freedberg, 1984).

In accordance with the Judeo-Christian ideals of good citizenship, upper- and middle-class female volunteers acted as "friendly visitors" who, through face-to-face contact, attempted to uplift the mental and moral nature of the less fortunate and to motivate people applying for aid to find decent work and become good citizens. It was the visitor's role to determine the worthiness of the dependent's character and needs through the relationship. Boston COS leader Octavia Hill's (1875) motto "not alms but a friend" was reflected in the charity worker's new attitude of sympathy, rather than fear and pity, toward the poor and the adverse circumstances they had to overcome.

While visitors were instructed to form friendly relations with the applicants, the disparity in social and economic power perpetuated a system of inherent paternalism that rendered the notion of "honest and simple" friendship somewhat paradoxical. The realization that the relations between visitor and client might not actually be "friendly," in the sense that they did not produce a basis for a satisfactory relationship, contributed to the decline of friendly visiting in the twentieth century and the move toward a more systematic method of helping the poor (Lubove, 1969). By the end of the 1800s, paid agents (usually men) had joined the ranks of the friendly visitors (usually women), and their strategies could be grouped into five areas representing the principles of what they called "scientific philanthropy": (1) investigation, (2) registration, (3) friendly visiting, (4) cooperation, and (5) constructive work. The major method of the Societies became systematic investigation into the causes of dependence and pauperism in order to provide an individualized solution to the problems of the poor.

As the nineteenth century drew to a close, charity giving was becoming more systematic and rational, heralding a new era of professionalism. With the rise of capitalism, guided by the American belief in "pulling yourself up by your own bootstraps," the notion of "rugged individualism" reflected the mood and culture of the country in this historical period. At this point in the profession's history, the caseworker's array of interventive tools was aimed at the individual, and the method of helping the poor based on one-to-one work with individuals served as the underpinning for the casework method.

The principle of individualizing poor and dependent clients was seen as progressive for the times, because it personalized the relationship and required that the worker accept and respect each individual client (Germain & Gitterman, 1996). This concern with individualization undercut the tendency toward moral judgment and the categorization of clients.

The recognition of the client–worker relationship as a key dynamic in social work practice was beginning to emerge through the work and writings of Mary Richmond. However, no scientific basis existed for understanding the effects of family relationships and complex interactions between and among individuals.

The professionalization of social work

Mary Richmond (1861–1928), a pioneer in the development of this new profession, helped shape American social work philosophy and practice during this period. By the turn of the twentieth century Richmond was established as a leader in the field, having been at the helm of two of the larger COSs in the country: the Baltimore Charity Organization Society (1891–1907) and the Philadelphia Charity Organization Society (1900–1905).

From the beginning of her career with the COS movement, Richmond recognized that the client–worker relationship itself was a fundamental factor in the helping process. According to Richmond (1899, p. 180), "Friendly visiting means intimate and continuous knowledge of and sympathy with a poor family's joys, sorrows, opinions, feelings, and entire outlook upon life." Clearly, Richmond was aware that the intention of the friendly visitor to "do good work" would have a relational impact on the client–worker relationship. However, she did not have a psychological framework to guide her practice; nor was there theory to help the worker understand the psychosocial dynamics intrinsic to relational processes. But this notion of the client–worker relationship was soon to transform itself into a more "professional" one, in which the worker used him or herself as an instrument for change.

By 1908, Richmond had moved away from her COS colleagues, whose focus had been on the moral roots of dependency, to a new concept of social work based on what she thought was a "scientific" approach to casework. In 1909 she became the director of the Russell Sage Foundation's Charity Organization Department in New York, where she was able to devote herself to writing, research, and the pedagogy of social casework (Pumphrey & Pumphrey, 1961).

Convinced that social work needed specific skills, knowledge, and a systematic method of practice that could be transmitted through formal training, Richmond called for the establishment of a school of "applied philanthropy." This was revolutionary because at this time women were not encouraged to undertake higher education in preparation for a paid career (Lubove, 1969). A one-year course was established at the New York School of Philanthropy in 1904 (later the New York School of Social Work, and since 1962, the Columbia University School of Social Work). Coinciding with the proliferation of schools of social work in pre-World War I America, the term "social worker" came into general usage (Ehrenreich, 1985).

Mary Richmond, like her contemporaries Mary Jarrett, a pioneering psychiatric social worker, and Ida Canon, an early medical social worker, recognized the importance of introducing a care-centered female relational field within a scientific framework of professional practice, both to legitimize themselves with respect to their client population, and to gain support from the male-dominated professions of medicine, psychology, and the natural sciences (Hiersteiner & Peterson, 1999). However, resistance to becoming involved in university education emanated, in part, from the Charity Movement's fear that greater emphasis on theory and method might dilute the visitor's charitable concern and helpfulness (Hiersteiner & Peterson, 1999).

Nevertheless, Richmond forged ahead in her efforts to professionalize social casework. Closely allied with the medical establishment in the Baltimore hospitals, she applied the linear model of the medical sciences to social casework, the dominant method of social work in her time. In her groundbreaking book *Social Diagnosis* (1917), she introduced her method of casework practice, arguing that good social work was based on disciplined study and observation, a thorough gathering of social evidence, an interpretation of the data, an accurate diagnosis of the problem, and an appropriate treatment plan. By demanding a thorough and systematic gathering of facts, she believed, the social worker could uncover the cause of the problem and develop an eventual "cure" for the person in trouble (Germain, 1970).

Implicit in this innovative approach to casework practice was her appreciation of relational ties in diagnosing personal difficulties. Richmond described "social diagnosis" as:

the attempt to make as exact a definition as possible of the situation and personality of a human being in some social need—of his situation and personality, that is, in relation to the other human beings upon whom he in any way depends or who depended upon him, and in relation to the social institutions of his community.

(Richmond, 1917, p. 357)

By the time she had written *Social Diagnosis*, Richmond (1917) had moved toward replacing the "friendly" relationship with the more formal expertise of a professional social worker trained in a systematic method of uncovering causes and treating the individual and family (Lubove, 1969). Her interpretation of social evidence gave her a better understanding of the social environment and her stress on "the action of mind upon mind" directed her attention toward the individual and his or her unique personal characteristics (Germain, 1970, p. 101).

What appeared to be missing from Richmond's social casework method was an analysis of complex interactions and relational dynamics and theories from which interventive methods could be derived. However, it must be kept in mind that at this point in time general acceptance of psychodynamic theories and relational concepts had not yet occurred.

By the 1920s the "friendly" relationship of the volunteer charity workers had been, by and large, replaced by the more formal expertise of the professional social worker trained in the systematic and thorough method of gathering extensive evidence, uncovering causes, and treating the individual and family based upon the social diagnosis.

In her book *What is Social Casework* (1922), Richmond continued to highlight the individualized approach to social work, focusing on the client's ability to adjust to the objective realities of life. She defined the casework method as consisting of "those processes which develop personality through adjustments consciously effected, individual by individual, between men and their social environments" (pp. 98–99). Social evidence provided a good deal of insight into the person and the problem; and although she considered the impact of the social context on the individual—family, friends, neighbors, and social institutions—her actual practice side-stepped social reform and was aimed squarely at individual change to increase the person's ability to adjust and function in the social environment.

This idea of the caseworker as a sympathetic "friend" and listener was developing into one in which the worker used him/herself as a disciplined instrument of change in Richmond's casework method. Professional spontaneity and warmth were compromised as the relationship resembled one in which clinical distance and logical thought dominated. Presumably, this more objective stance would allow the worker to maintain enough objectivity to gather evidence, categorize questions, and organize information elicited in order to make the best social diagnosis possible.

Interestingly, case material cited in *What is Social Casework* reflected the way in which the worker used him/herself was similar to contemporary practice skills and techniques, such as active listening, reflection, exploration. Richmond cites an example in which a client was talking about problems she was having with her mother. In order for the worker to be fair and objective, she/he needed to help the client see both sides of the situation. The worker said: "From what I have heard, I do not think you have told me everything. This led to a quite different account which was possible to substantiate later." The worker's attention to the client's relationship with her mother presages the profession's future concern with relational issues.

Like the friendly visitor of the COS, the social worker remained in control of the relationship. The difference was that in Richmond's configuration, the client was viewed as a diagnostic entity dependent on the social worker who, armed with expert knowledge, used him or herself as a professional tool to effect change within the individual (Ehrenreich, 1985).

However, it is important to note that, compared to the preconceived moral judgments about the character of the poor held by early COS workers, Richmond's objective approach to problem solving, which individualized each client's particular situation, was progressive for her time. The establishment of a professional client–caseworker relationship required objectivity; there was no room for moral judgment (Lubove, 1969).

The Settlement House era: late nineteenth to early twentieth centuries

Simultaneously with the COS movement, the Settlement House movement began in large cities at the turn of the twentieth century when social work was in transition from an avocation to a paid profession; it was a time when thousands of immigrants were arriving in America daily, looking for opportunities and freedom in a newly prospering society. However, for the newcomers, housing, working conditions, and sanitary conditions were poor, and immigrants making substandard wages were forced to crowd into steamy tenements and city streets.

The settlement workers were mostly middle-class, educated young men and women, who sought to carry out their mission in close relation to the people they served. Unlike Richmond's early caseworkers, these dedicated settlers established relationships that involved doing with, rather than doing for, with the intention of promoting equality between themselves and community residents.

Concerned about the inequities they witnessed, they believed that living among the community residents in poor and working-class neighborhoods would bring about a level of relational intimacy that would be beneficial in raising their neighbors' sense of cultural, political, social, and intellectual awareness. The personal relationships that the settlers attempted to develop with neighborhood residents was an attempt to reduce social distance in the interest of working together toward common goals of economic and social justice (Specht, 1994).

The settlers believed in what Jane Addams, prominent reformer and Settlement House pioneer, called the "reciprocal relationship of classes" (Addams, 1960). Concerned that these newcomers, who had virtually little or no political power, could be manipulated for the good of local politicians, they engaged in progressive political activities and were in the vanguard of many reform efforts, such as public health, education, and vocational training (Beck, 1977).

Addams and the other settlers saw the newcomers as alienated and disconnected from their new society. They perceived their work as a way to help the immigrants feel less anonymous and more connected to the other people and institutions in their neighborhood. By working side by side with community residents, and through close participation in the neighborhood life and community relations, settlement workers believed they could advance the best interests of the local residents. In their helping relationships, they modeled appropriate social roles, helped immigrants adapt to American ways, and worked to develop interpersonal relationships into a mutual aid system (Wenocur & Reisch, 1989).

Furthermore, Addams, who believed that women should be active in community and political affairs, also saw settlement work as an outlet for women to extend their natural sense of maternal responsibility—the skills and values of motherhood—to disenfranchised and economically disadvantaged communities. Ironically, gender roles traditionally associated with the domestic sphere replicated themselves in relationships outside the home, perpetuating gender-linked stereotypes associated with the social work profession (Ehrenreich, 1985).

The Settlement House commitment to instructional and practical services, group activities, and social reform was the forerunner of the group work method of the 1930s, 1940s, and 1950s and the community action movement of the 1960s. Regardless of the specific approach—developmental, rehabilitative, recreational, or mutual aid—the group worker's prevailing consideration was to elicit common concerns, common interests, and common life situations, and to instigate group interaction so that members felt invested in each other and in the group. Boundaries between leader and group varied depending on the type of group, although the original premise of group work was to encourage a democratic process of group involvement, which means that the main source of growth resides within the member and their interactions with each other (Tropp, 1977).

The impact of Freud on social casework

Before World War I, social work had little awareness of Sigmund Freud, whose psychoanalytic theory had not strongly established itself on American soil. His theory began to receive widespread attention at a time when returning World War I veterans were suffering from war neurosis. A need for psychiatrically trained social workers provided the impetus behind the opening of the Smith College Training School for Psychiatric Social Workers in 1918.

By the 1920s and 1930s, Freud's theory of personality development had become increasingly influential in social work circles, especially in understanding problems of maladjustment with a newly emerging middle-class clientele. Social workers now had a theoretical framework through which to analyze unconscious inner needs, individual problems, and root causes of behavior heretofore missing from Richmond's sociologically oriented casework. Problems were defined in personality terms resulting from intrapsychic conflicts that often were projected onto interpersonal functioning and relational issues.

Analytic theory may have restricted social work's focus on issues within the psyche and inner life of the client rather than the individual in relation to others, but it also brought attention to the importance of family relationships and the client–worker relationship. With regard to familial relational patterns, Freud constructed his psychosexual theory on the impact of the child's relational patterns with both mother and father (Hollis, 1964). Freud's analysis of the patient's relationship with the mother as the primary object for instinctually driven needs during the first four years of life was a key factor in shaping the future personality of the child. Another critical issue, according to Freud, that impacts on personality development, includes the growing child's awakening genital fantasies of sexual union with the parent of the opposite sex. This awareness creates anxiety for fear of retaliation from the desired parental figure.

The resolution of this conflict, which Freud calls the Oedipal complex for the boy, and the Electra complex for the girl, lies in the boy's renunciation of sexual feelings for the mother, and the girl's renunciation of sexual feelings for the father. The original Oedipal fantasies are repressed, and replaced by love and admiration for the mother by the boy and the father by the girl. Thus, a relationship with the parent figure is built on respect and a desire for reciprocal love. The result of this drama is that the relational bonds, which get replayed throughout one's life, are intense and central to the psychosexual development of the individual (Brenner, 1974).

At that time clinicians were becoming aware that a positive therapeutic relationship facilitated the patient's disclosure of personal material, making possible a more accurate diagnosis and treatment plan (Turner, 2002). The concept of transference was of particular relevance to Freud and his followers. Transference phenomena—feelings and thoughts clients had toward earlier significant figures in their lives that they unconsciously attributed to the worker—may emerge at any point in a relationship with the worker (Turner, 2002). Most social workers, knowing that these irrational feelings were merely symbolic of relationships with other persons in their past or present life, were cautioned not to interpret or encourage transference material (Perlman, 1957). However, a small group of psychoanalytically trained caseworkers believed that understanding the meaning of transferential material could provide the key that unlocked neurotic conflicts. Providing clients with insight into these emotional processes could help them see how they repeated these relational patterns in the present (Garrett, 1958).

Freudian thinkers conceived of the individual psyche as an isolated entity only modestly influenced by the social group, its structures and processes. His model of the therapeutic relationship encouraged the worker to maintain an impassive self with rigid ego boundaries. Further, this relationship was cast as one-directional, leaving the social worker in control of the destiny of his or her clients. Whereas social work increasingly began to regard effective social functioning as integral to its success, psychoanalytic theory directed the practitioner's interest more narrowly toward resolving conflicts and individual problems, leading the worker toward a form of practice directly removed from the community (Agnew, 2004). Analytic theory may have narrowed social work's interest to issues within the individual psyche and the inner life of the client rather than the individual in relation to others, but it did bring attention to the importance of the client–worker relationship and relationships within the family in clinical practice.

The diagnostic school

The impact of Freudian psychoanalysis on social work theory in the 1920s and 1930s contributed to the development of the diagnostic school of social casework practice associated with such eminent scholar–practitioners as Gordon Hamilton, Fern Lowry, Lucille Austin, Annette Garrett, Betsey Libbey, and Grace Marcus (Minahan, 1986; Smalley, 1970). This phase of social work philosophy and practice, which spanned two world wars, was called the diagnostic school because of its stress on the importance of diagnosis in the treatment process. The diagnostic school furthered the development of casework as the dominant method in the field by giving it a theoretical base.

The diagnostic school viewed the therapeutic process as goal-directed and based upon the client's personality factors and social situation. The worker took responsibility for gathering data and evaluating individual capacities and limitations in order to arrive at therapeutic goals. Thus, on the basis of understanding the psychodynamics of the case, together with an assessment of the client's psychological status, the nature of the client's problems, and the social situation, a psychosocial diagnosis became the basis for intervention.

Fern Lowry elaborated on the concept of diagnosis and criticized the trend toward viewing history, diagnosis, and treatment as time-fixed facts in the life of a case. She visualized it as a more dynamic concept weaving in and out of treatment. Still viewed as a thinking process aimed at better understanding and treating the client's problem, it became even clearer that the therapeutic relationship was integral to diagnosis as a process. Practitioners were aware that as the relationship developed, and as more material from the client's life unfolded, it was easier to adjust earlier diagnostic formulations throughout the life of the treatment process (Finlayson, 1937).

In a manner similar to that of Mary Richmond, the diagnostic school of social workers viewed the relationship as a means through which clinicians found new ways of looking at themselves and their problems. This process was enhanced by a supportive worker, who could motivate the client toward accomplishing the treatment goal that best met the client's particular needs and diagnosis. The worker was there to listen and understand, and to help the client share life experiences and feelings in a way that might result in a reduction of tension and anxiety (Casius, 1950).

The functional school

During the late 1930s and early 1940s, a schism developed between caseworkers who adhered to the diagnostic school and those who followed the functional approach to casework practice, which was based on Otto Rank's concept of the will. Rank placed particular emphasis on the individual will—a controlling, organizing force in the personality—and used this concept of will as a substitute for the ego (Smalley, 1970).

Perhaps as a result of the sense of helplessness that many social workers felt during the Great Depression, Rank's optimistic view of humankind was much welcomed in the post-Depression era. The intent of the functional social worker was to move away from a deterministic Freudian interpretation of behavior in which the person was seen as driven by instinctual forces, to one in which the individual was deemed more in control of his or her life. Individuals' inborn will naturally moved them from an initial state of seeking union with significant others toward a state of individuation and autonomy in which they could eventually take over their own problem solving processes.

Rank's theory of personality and behavior held particular appeal for social worker Virginia Robinson and psychologist Dr. Jesse Taft, faculty members at the University of Pennsylvania School of Social Work, who saw the client–worker relationship as the core to all clinical processes. Rather than trying to achieve any predetermined end based on an initial diagnosis as in the diagnostic school, the functional school worker used the relationship as a tool to help clients realize their own potential and reach psychological equilibrium (Robinson, 1930). According to Robinson, "engaging the other" through a professional social work relationship could release the growth potential inherent in all human beings, enabling clients to make and act on choices or decisions they identified as their own. The functionalists focused on the client's current situation as reflected in the relationship with the social worker who carried out the function of the social work agency. The worker's use of agency function and structure and the purpose of the services being offered directed the helping process (Casius, 1950; Smalley, 1970).

In her landmark book *A Changing Psychology in Social Casework* (1930), Robinson championed the use of the social work relationship as the primary tool of the social worker involved in a casework process oriented toward helping people make use of agency services in constructive ways (Smalley, 1970). The social worker's competence and skills depended to a great degree on his/her own self-development and self-awareness. The client's ability to engage in a growth-promoting relationship with a mature, self-aware worker could then be transferred to real-life situations in which new patterns of interacting with people in the environment could be established.

The following vignette illustrates how the diagnostic and functional approaches may be applied to practice. Mr. and Mrs. A came to a family service agency because of problems they were having with their 10-year-old daughter, Janine. Janine, the eldest of four girls, was having the hardest time with the fact that her mother had breast cancer 18 months ago. Although her mother is now cancer free, Janine was very anxious about leaving Mrs. A and frequently refused to go to school. The diagnostic caseworker gathered as much information as possible on past history and present behavior in order to shed more light on the reasons for Janine's anxiety. The worker perceived that the underlying cause of Janine's problematic behavior was her separation anxiety, since these symptoms surfaced when her mother was diagnosed with cancer. The caseworker sought to gain a clearer understanding of the specifics of the mother–child relationship, the parents' attitude toward Mrs. A's illness, their relationship, and Janine's early development, first by taking a history and then through observation. With the caseworker's support and understanding, the therapeutic intervention began with enabling Janine to talk about her fears and concerns about her mother's health. The worker was also concerned that Mr. and Mrs. A may be transferring their own anxiety onto Janine and met with them separately to help them talk about their feelings about the state of Mrs. A's health.

A social worker guided by the functional approach would spend more time reviewing agency services and function than gathering a family history and developmental history of Janine. For example, the agency provides family counseling, family advocacy, and family-life education. The worker would contract with the client system and would help Janine and her parents decide how they can best utilize these services and how they think they can benefit from the casework relationship. The social worker's activities might be directed toward helping the parents become better informed and self-directing so that they themselves can take more responsibility in helping Janine get to school. The worker models developmentally appropriate ways for Mr. and Mrs. A to deal with Janine in the here-and-now.

The schism between the functional and diagnostic schools became more pronounced in the 1930s, when functional casework challenged Freudian concepts of therapy and placed its emphasis on time limited treatment goals. The functional school rejected the diagnostic school's emphasis on extensive fact gathering and a worker-focus diagnosis and treatment plan. Instead, they believed that the relationship process could provide clients with an opportunity to release growth potential and exercise choice in such a way that the client was free to accept or reject the agency's service.

Nevertheless, even though the functional school of thought emphasized a more or less linear model of assessment, the two approaches had more in common than their adherents may have realized. In both schools the worker controlled the relationship by virtue of either agency function or worker diagnosis.

Development of relational perspective after World War II

After World War II, American social work philosophy and practice shifted toward what would now be called a "relational" perspective. In the late 1940s and the 1950s, efforts were made to bridge the gap between the functionalists and diagnostics, and greater attention was paid to clients' interactions with the social systems in their environment. Adapting psychodynamic ideas to a more social concept of casework, a group of eminent social work scholars and practitioners from the pre-war era, including Gordon Hamilton, Bertha Capen Reynolds, Florence Hollis, and Helen Harris Perlman, were instrumental in shaping the new American social work philosophy and practice.

An adherent of the diagnostic school, Gordon Hamilton saw the client–worker relationship as a way to strengthen and assess the individual's capacity to take action in relation to the environment. She expanded social work's unit of attention beyond the individual to include the impinging environment and the problem situation, which she termed the "person-in-situation configuration" (Germain, 1970; Hamilton, 1951). Reacting to the caseworker's bias toward the psychological aspects of practice, Hamilton's person-in-situation paradigm was an attempt to view both the inner psychological realities and the objective social context as one interrelated whole (Germain, 1970).

For Hamilton, the concept of human relationships was fundamental to social casework practice: the experience of having a friendly, interested worker listen attentively to one's troubles, not minimize the difficulty, not criticize or advise, tended to induce a warm response in the client leading to a sense of being understood—the deepest bond in either a personal or a professional association (Hamilton, 1951). Like Mary Richmond, Hamilton emphasized the fact that the worker must individualize all aspects of the casework relationship. For example, two pregnant teenage mothers may be facing the same economic and family difficulties, yet each might react differently to her situation. Thus the social worker reacts differently as well. Or two pregnant teenage mothers may react in similar ways but be facing different economic and family difficulties

Helen Harris Perlman, noted for her problem-solving method, examined the significance of the role of the helping relationship in the casework process. She writes about the client–worker relationship:

> it is a means of communication between two people involved in treatment; it is a set of attitudes and a set of responses expressed in behavior. When both individuals in the casework relationship interact with warmth, acceptance, and feeling, energy is freed up generating the motivation toward problem solving and the use of help.
>
> (Perlman, 1957, p. 149)

The relationship can also serve as a corrective mechanism where social workers are trained to be aware of their reactions, to control their responses, and to act in a way that demonstrates good will and warmth toward the client. She states that "relationship is a human being's feeling or sense of bonding with another" (Perlman, 1979, p. 23). Influenced by concepts drawn from ego psychology, Perlman noted that one of the purposes of the helping relationship is to help people exercise their own problem-solving capacities in coping with their lives. This involves helping people to think for themselves and encouraging clients to utilize their strengths in such as way as to best adapt to their environment.

Perhaps more than anyone, Bertha Capen Reynolds, a practitioner, scholar, and activist, recognized the interdependence between the client and his or her social community. Having witnessed the erosion of democratic values and individual freedoms in Europe, she asserted the importance of establishing a social work relationship that made it possible to maximize a sense of equality and mutuality between client and worker. Reynolds's perspective on relationships was as much a political and philosophical orientation as it was a practice principle. Delivering social work services in the Personal Social Service Department of the United Seamen's Service, she believed that because both client and worker were members of the same organization, a reciprocal relationship between the two was possible.

The Personal Social Service Department, situated in the hall of the National Maritime Union, made it possible for Reynolds to work in close proximity to the people social work served. Consistent with her democratic philosophy, she placed the principle of client self-determination—the client's right to determine his or her own course of treatment—in the center of the social work process, freeing clients from the vestiges of a paternalistic relationship (Reynolds, 1951).

In the 1950s and 1960s, borrowing concepts from social systems theory and the ecological perspective, clinicians became increasingly aware of the ways in which individuals were engaged in constant exchanges with other social systems in their environment. According to Germain and Gitterman, the ecological perspective, and its adaptive view of people and their environments, led clinicians to seek to understand how each acts and influences the other: "Human relatedness is a biological and social imperative for the human being over the life span. Without relationships the human infant cannot survive, and without relatedness the human being cannot learn to be human" (1986, p. 621).

These ideas led the profession to pay greater attention to clients' interaction with others: the development of social networks, concepts of relatedness, competence, and self-esteem. Ego psychology seemed to be the bridge that could link individuals to their social environments. According to Eda Goldstein (1984), ego psychology comprises a related set of theoretical concepts about human behavior that focus on the origins, development, structure, and functioning of the executive arm of the personality—the ego. The ego is considered to be a mental structure of the personality that is responsible for negotiating the internal needs of the individual with the outside world. Ego psychology helped clinicians focus on the individual's adaptive capacities to cope with internal and external stress, and to form and sustain healthy relationships.

Florence Hollis, a leader in the field of psychosocial casework in the 1950s, seemed to understand that the task of casework was to help people learn to adjust more effectively to their social situations. In her book *Casework: A Psychosocial Therapy* (1981), Hollis focused on the "treatment of individuals experiencing problems in their interpersonal relationships" (p. 3). Hollis viewed the client–worker relationship as a microcosm through which to assess the difficulties clients might be having in other relationships in their lives. She emphasized the importance of the continuous interaction between inner psychological processes and external social systems. In essence, Hollis elaborated on Hamilton's person-in-situation configuration to frame her psychosocial approach to casework.

In spite of the expanded explanations of the psychosocial realities of people's lives, the vast majority of writings on casework were still closely connected to the casework tradition of individual diagnosis and treatment. Interventions were still basically targeted at personality change, perhaps because influencing social relationships was a political issue that agencies did not have the power or authority to address (Germain, 1970).

In the 1960s, however, large-scale social change impacted the social work field and redirected attention to the social environment. The War on Poverty, the Economic Opportunity Act of 1964, the civil rights movement, and later movements for equality such as the women's movement inspired the launching of community action programs. These programs emphasized concrete services such as day care and health services, along with community participation, group methods, and advocacy. Community representatives were invited to sit on agency boards in policy-making and advisory roles, and sometimes were involved in planning and administering programs (Germain & Gitterman, 1986).

Practice models in the 1960s and 1970s recognized the need of oppressed groups to feel a sense of empowerment in their relationships with others and in relation to the economic, political, and social realities of their lives. According to Goldstein et al. (2009), empowerment approaches attempted to improve clients' self-esteem, by giving them a sense of personal control over their lives. Also, these programs fostered collaboration in the client–worker relationship and the belief that individuals could have an impact on others and their communities.

Since the 1960s, social work has ventured in new directions, incorporating new theoretical and practical approaches best suited to the populations served, while remaining true to the purpose and values of its professional foundation. These new concepts and techniques include family theory and family therapy, crisis theory and crisis intervention, task-centered short-term work, cognitive behavior approaches, self-help groups, and cultural and cross-cultural theories, psychodynamic relational concepts, and relational–cultural theory.

Relational–cultural theory seeks to integrate the person (inner psyche) and environment (external events), guiding the clinical process of assessment and intervention toward the interpersonal realm of people's lives. It has grown from the early work of Jean Baker Miller's self-in-relation theory (see Miller, 1976) to include the impact of socio-cultural concepts on assessment and intervention. Its tenets, practice interventions, and knowledge base are shaped by social structures and power arrangements that circumscribe the role of women and men.

2   Relational theory in a nutshell

When a profession incorporates a new theoretical framework, it is important to understand the theoretical roots and building blocks upon which new concepts and clinical applications are based. Relational–cultural theory (RCT) builds upon basic concepts drawn from psychodynamic relational theory, interpersonal theory, object relations theory, self-psychology, ego psychology—all subsumed in this chapter under the rubric of relational theories. Notable theorists representing these schools include Robert Stolorow, Erik Erikson, John Bowlby, Heinz Kohut, Harry Stack Sullivan, Otto Kernberg, Nancy Chodorow, and Carol Gilligan—each relational to some degree and each representing a shift from the Freudian individualistic model of psychosexual development toward a model which views relationship as both the process and goal of human development (Miller, 1976; Miller & Stiver, 1997; Walker, 2004).

These approaches, while differing in some aspects, share the following features: (1) an emphasis on the individual's developing sense of self, the belief that connective and affiliative needs are crucial to growth and development of the self; and (2) an emphasis on the interaction between the individual and the object world—that is, the nature and qualities of this interaction with others as predictors of personality development, psychosocial functioning, and change.

The relational–cultural perspective, which frames the case illustrations in this book, offers a new concept of the nature of the self. It is a body of work that highlights the significance of interpersonal relationships. Relational theorists, especially during the last three decades, have paid increasing attention to the mutual influence of clients and clinicians, as well as the nature and quality of relational matrixes in clients' lives.

Klein and Horney

The early roots of the relational–cultural perspective can be found in the work of Melanie Klein and Karen Horney, two female psychoanalysts writing and practicing in the 1920s, 1930s and 1940s. Neo-Freudians in their own right, they revised Freud's theory that presented a picture of human beings motivated by id-driven drives and needs in which the primary goal of behavior is the attainment of gratification and the reduction of tension. In this psychoanalytic model, the self is shaped not by mutually interacting relationships with others, but by relating to the other as an object whose sole purpose is to satiate one's impulses and gratify one's needs.

As female psychoanalysts, Klein and Horney understood the shortcomings of applying Freudian theory to female patients, and interpreted psychoanalytic conflict within an interpersonal and cultural context. Although Klein and Horney gradually gained acceptance in the male-oriented psychiatric world of the 1920s and 1930s, and made major contributions to understanding human behavior and development, they were not widely known in mainstream social work circles.

The British object relations theorist Melanie Klein's concept of object-related drive theory emerged in the 1930s and expanded on Freud's drive model (Greenberg & Mitchell, 1983). Building on Freud's view that the infant is driven by basic biological imperatives and drives, she broadened its scope to include the object world (that is, other people). Klein understood that drives were inherently connected to a complex web of objects in the environment, and, therefore, intrinsically relational (St. Clair & Wigren, 2004).

Klein used the term *inner object* to suggest that the infant internalizes the object in the outer world—that being the mother or primary caretaker—and identifies with that object as if they were one and the same from birth. In fact the infant's internalized sense of self is not made up of the actual characteristics of the real external object, but rather the infant's fantasy about his/her imagined relationship to the mother figure. In this way, Klein believed that it was the infant's own mental processes and need for relatedness to another person that linked him/her to others at the earliest moments of life (St. Clair & Wigren, 2004; Goldstein, 2001).

Klein's understanding of the inner world of the child gives insight into early dyadic relational processes, and provides a window through which to look into later relational conflicts and processes. However, while Klein attributed fundamental importance to the infant's first object relation—the mother's breast—feminist relational theorists note that object relational needs are central throughout the life cycle. In Klein's view, the quality of interpersonal relationships experienced by the infant is crucial to the child's ability to master appropriate developmental stages and becomes the basis for personality development.

Karen Horney, a contemporary of Melanie Klein, cast relational processes beyond the dyadic encounter to include the larger social and cultural context. A critic of Freud's view of female sexuality, she challenged the well-accepted assumption of penis envy popular in the mainstream psychoanalytic circles of her time. Rather than ascribe any sense of "envy" to a biological fate of circumstance, she attributed women's feelings of inferiority to their social subordination in an inherently male-dominated culture. It is not the male anatomical apparatus that women want, Horney asserted, but rather the access to what men have: power, opportunity, and resources (Berzoff et al., 2011).

According to Horney, libido was still biological, but any sense of anatomical inferiority resulted from a realistic appraisal of the power structure of social relations in the real world. "If a little boy is adored by his family, his sister wants what he has, not the anatomical [thing] but the emotional gratification he experiences" (Lacan, 1985, p. 125). Thus, Horney shifted the focus of female problems from a biologically and sexually rooted neurosis to a concern with the psycho-social context of interpersonal relations.

The Interpersonal School

About a decade after Horney and Klein presented their socio-cultural view of psycho-analytic theory, Harry Stack Sullivan challenged Freud's focus on instinctual drives and individual processes, concentrating on the interpersonal context within which personality is shaped and behavior takes place. Sullivan's work on interpersonal relationships became the foundation of interpersonal psychoanalysis, a school of psychoanalytic theory and treatment that stresses the detailed exploration of the nuances of patients' patterns of interacting with others.

Sullivan defined personality as "the relatively enduring pattern of recurrent interpersonal situations which characterize a human life" (Sullivan, 1940, p. xi). For example, he posited that behavior which may seem meaningless when viewed as an individual response will take on new meaning when observed in an interpersonal context such as the family. In other words, according to Sullivan, personality does not reside in the individual mind. Rather, the relational matrix—past and present relationships—is the organizer of the self and gives root to the development of personality (Goldstein et al., 2009).

Sullivan's approach does not discount nature or heredity as having an impact on personality; the human brain and one's genetic predispositions develop in tandem with social and cultural experiences, minimizing binary pulls toward nature or nurture (Mitchell, 1988). The child is not a blank slate, and each individual reacts to different situations with his/her unique responses. However, the individual is clearly a product of interaction with other human beings, and it is the interactional field, not the individual mind, that is the unit for the study of emotional life and where clinical interventions take place.

As Sullivan developed his approach, he increasingly focused on anxiety as the motivating force in the way the individual shapes his or her experiences in the world (Mitchell & Black, 1995). For example, if anxiety is present in the "mothering" of the infant, the young child will look for a secure base in another to reduce the tension associated with the anxiety that the nurturing figure has induced. Subsequently, interactions that an individual experiences as painful or threatening will continue to drive behavior as the individual avoids situations based on previous interpersonal experiences. On the other hand, social interaction that provides a secure base can lead to a lessening of anxiety within the individual. For Sullivan, the personal relationship between therapist and patient can serve as a corrective emotional experience and is an important determining factor in the outcome of treatment.

Sullivan's belief that the self is constituted through relationships with others is an important forerunner of the self-in-relation theory that originated at the Stone Center for Developmental Services and Studies. He reaffirmed the belief that the human being is inextricably linked to others in a series of interpersonal fields and that the need for soothing social relations continues to evolve throughout the life cycle. It is important to note here that the objective reality of one person's experience with another is often not as important as what this experience subjectively means to the client (Mitchell & Black, 1995). The issues presented to the clinician are: what kind of human interactions keep the person locked into nonproductive habits, and what can be done to change these patterns?

Ego psychology

Ego psychology represented a more optimistic, growth-oriented view of human functioning than did earlier deterministic theories such as Freudian psychology. Ego psychologists such as Anna Freud, Heinz Hartmann, and Erik Erikson emphasized the ego's rational and unconscious capacities to adapt to environmental factors and the capacity for growth and change throughout the life cycle (Goldstein, 1984).

Eda Goldstein, a prominent social work educator and clinician, introduced the theory and practice of ego psychology to students, educators, and practitioners in her well-known book *Ego Psychology and Social Work Practice* (1984). The application of ego psychology led to changes in the assessment process and interventive strategies, resulting in a renewed emphasis upon work with the family, group, and other significant individuals in the social and physical environment. Clinicians who use an ego psychological approach are concerned with the individual's adaptation to the external world as well as with the quality of interpersonal relationships.

The ego contains the basic functions essential to the individual's successful adaptation to the environment. Object (or interpersonal) relations is one of the twelve ego functions identified by Leopold Bellak and his colleagues that is of primary interest to relational theorists. It refers to the quality of one's interpersonal relationships and the ability to sustain and form stable relationships with others with a minimum of hostility and frustration (Bellak & Goldsmith, 1984).

Erik Erikson, a major contributor to ego psychology, had a considerable impact on clinical theory and practice. He departed from Freud's drive theory by introducing a series of constructs that emphasized the interactional aspects of ego development. Like Harry Stack Sullivan before him, Erikson highlighted the importance of interpersonal relationships in shaping personality.

Erikson described ego development as involving progressive mastery of developmental tasks in each of eight successive stages throughout the life cycle. In his formulation, each stage presents the individual with an associated normative life crisis and specific psychological and social tasks to master (Goldstein, 1996).

In each successive stage of Erikson's developmental model, the social radius of significant relationships changes and widens. For example, in infancy, the first stage of life, the crucial figures with whom the infant interacts, and who are central to satisfying the task of developing a sense of trust in him or herself and in the object world, are the primary caregivers. As the infant develops and moves into young childhood, relationships with schoolmates, neighborhood friends, and teachers become significant figures in meeting the bio-psycho-social needs attendant to each successive stage of development.

While this paradigm implies that the ideal resolution of later phases is dependent on previous ones, Erikson's orientation allows for the reworking of earlier tasks with individuals in the social environment. His concept of the developing self in relation to others paved the way for relational elements to filter into social work's theory and practice base.

The object relations school

Beginning in the 1940s and 1950s, the emerging British and American object relations school of psychology gained popularity in the social sciences and contributed to social work's understanding of people's adaptation to the social environment and interpersonal relations with the object world. The term "object," a technical word originally coined by Freud to refer simply to "that which will satisfy a need," was broadened to refer to the significant person or thing that is the object or target of another's feelings or drives (St. Clair & Wigren, 2004).

Another use of the term object relations refers to specific intrapsychic structures, an aspect of ego organization that is developed in relation to the infant's inner representation of self in relation to others. The study of the internal and external world of object relations suggests that subjective, internalized images of significant persons, usually mother, father, or primary caregiver, become more important in the formation and differentiation of self than the actual interactions. However, inner residues of past relationships with significant persons often become patterns that emerge in later experiences with others and exert a strong influence throughout life (St. Clair & Wigren, 2004).

Scottish psychoanalyst W.R.D. Fairbairn constructed a model of object relations that was perhaps more psychological and less biological than those of any of his neo-Freudian counterparts. In other words, his theory arose not from biologically based libidinal impulses as in Freud's drive model, but from the child striving for relationships with objects, specifically the primary caretakers. Fairbairn's developmental focus was on the nature of the object and the quality of the relationship (Mitchell, 1988).

Like Melanie Klein, Fairbairn believed that the ego and object are inseparable. Unlike Klein, he argued that the ego has its own source of energy, separate and apart from instinctual impulses, and organizes itself as a consequence of the accumulated quality of its relations with external objects during the first year of life. He argued further that the infant is oriented toward others from the beginning, not just to relieve bodily tensions and frustration, but to establish an emotional bond with an external object. Similar to Bowlby and other attachment theorists, the essential principle in Fairbairn's structural system is that the human being is essentially relation seeking. Propelled by its own source of energy, the self or ego seeks out and maintains an intensive emotional bond with an external object throughout life (Kernberg, 1976).

Typically, object relations theorists trace the trajectory of normal development as a movement from infantile dependence on a part object (one aspect of object is perceived, e.g. the mother's breast) to a mature dependence on a whole object (perception of object as a whole person). Growth moves from an infantile attitude of taking to a more mature attitude of mutual giving and receiving between two differentiated individuals (St. Clair & Wigren, 2004). The emphasis shifts from taking to giving, so that eventually a mutual exchange takes place.

Writing in the 1940s, 1950s, and 1960s, D.W. Winnicott represented a new voice in the British object relations school. He viewed the development of the self from a relational point of view, with special emphasis on understanding child development, especially the nature and quality of the mother–child interaction. Winnicott emphasized two key concepts that are relevant today to social work's dual focus on the person and environment: (1) the facilitating holding environment, with its emphasis on adaptation, and (2) the "good enough mother," with its focus on the proper parental attunement to the infant's needs and wants.

Winnicott linked the development of a healthy sense of self to specific qualities of this "good enough mother" (Mitchell, 1988). He invoked the idea of a reasonably empathic caregiver who is attuned to the infant's basic socio-emotional and survival needs. The "facilitating" environment provided by this "good enough" mother represents her effort to shape the environment around the child's wishes and to intuit what the child needs and wants. Winnicott places much importance on ego relatedness; primary relational experiences—feelings of belonging, of being understood, accepted, and loved—create the context for the development of self (Guntrip, 1971). Winnicott keeps the relationship in the spotlight, regardless of the intervention. However, like Klein, Winnicott's theories are anchored in Freud's instinctual model, in which pleasure from need-satisfaction forms the basis of relationship.

British psychoanalyst John Bowlby believed that individuals are motivated not by drives, but by forming attachments to other persons from the moment of birth. Bowlby devoted extensive research to the concept of attachment, describing it as a "lasting psychological connectedness between human beings" (Bowlby, 1969, p. 177). He proposed attachment theory as a way of understanding human beings' propensity to create strong emotional bonds to significant others and of explaining the many forms of personality disturbance and distress that occur after separation and loss. Bowlby shared the psychoanalytic view that early experiences in childhood have an important influence on development and behavior later in life. In Bowlby's theory, early attachment styles are established in childhood through the infant–caregiver relationship.

Similar to imprinting in the animal species, Bowlby believed that attachment had an evolutionary component in that it aided the survival function by enhancing safety through the infant's proximity to the caregiver (Bowlby, 1969). Drawing on a wide range of ethnological studies of instinctive behavior, Bowlby saw attachment as an inborn, instinctive mechanism that is ascendant in the earliest years, the most critical and vulnerable time in the infant's life: "The propensity to make strong emotional bonds to particular individuals [is] a basic component of human nature" (Bowlby, 1969, p. 3).

According to Bowlby, attachment motivates the child to move toward a caregiving figure for protection, warmth, nurturing, and social interaction, in addition to feeding. The psychological goal of proximity for survival is later supplanted by the more psychological goal of feeling close to the caregiver, whose responses strongly influence the child's present and future behavior patterns and personality states (Fonagy, 2001). Bowlby argued that the infant's attachment to the mother, or primary nurturing figure, is a precondition for the satisfaction of all other needs, making her a primary object of importance (Mitchell, 1988).

Infant developmental research

Any new theoretical paradigm for practice must rest on research-based propositions. Infant research has documented empirical evidence of Bowlby's theory of attachment as a drive. Infant researcher Daniel Stern (1985) provides empirical support for the idea that reciprocal interactions between mother and infant begin at birth, with each regulating their responses in anticipation of the other, jointly constructing interactive patterns that become organized over time. Infants bring with them a basic awareness of self that is shaped by ongoing interactions with the caretaking environment (Beebe & Lachmann, 2002).

In *The Interpersonal World of the Infant* (1985), Stern describes his research on the infant's subjective experiences, focusing on the interaction and mutual regulation of babies and their primary caretakers. He hypothesizes that the infant forms his or her subjective sense of self in relation to another from the very beginning of life. For example, at the end of the first week of life, Stern argues, the mother's face has become a familiar perceptual gestalt and the infant can distinguish the smell of his or her own mother from that of others, indicating that the infant can conceive of another person outside his or her self-boundaries. Each side of the mother–infant dyad complements the other; one person performs an action and the other receives it.

As a result of Stern's observations of newborns interacting with their primary caretakers, he proposed that the early formation of a sense of core self is developed during the first month of life. He infers that the infant does not enter the world in a state of undifferentiated fusion, as some object relations theorists believed, but rather that the infant comes into the world with a cognitive awareness of him or herself as distinct from others. Thus, Stern's organizing perspective places the relational self at the center of development from the moment the infant is born and asserts that this self is in a constant state of elaboration and reorganization throughout life.

According to Stern (1985), different senses of self emerge with the development of new capacities, the first being the core sense of self. At each major shift in maturation, there is a change in the subjective experience of the infant. For example, the infant takes part in regulating the level of excitement caused by the outside world by using gaze aversion to reduce stimulation that has risen above an optimum range. The caretaker, in turn, regulates his/her responses to adjust to the infant's stimulus barrier. With this kind of mutual regulation, the infant gains experience with self-regulation in response to the caregiver's sensitivities and ability to help the infant experience a greater sense of mastery over the environment (Fonagy, 2001).

Stern's work suggests that a major task for the individual is to create increasingly complex and intimate ties with others while at the same time perceiving him or herself as having a self that is separate from the other. In other words, the process of development does not involve merger at one pole versus differentiation at the other, but rather the ability to balance the development of a separate self with the awareness and experience of interacting with another that makes for a healthy personality (Fonagy, 2001).

Through repeated observations of mother–infant interactions, other infant–parent researchers, such as Beatrice Beebe and Frank Lachmann (2002), have also demonstrated that parent–child behavior does not operate in a unidirectional fashion. Rather it is a dyadic system characterized by mutual and reciprocal social exchanges over time. Each response by parent or infant triggers specific actions in the other, resulting in a continuous feedback loop (Brazelton et al., 1974). These interacting behaviors form patterns that may affect the nature of a person's relationships throughout life.

Self-psychology

Self-psychology, like other relational theories, rests on the premise that people have a powerful tendency to repeat basic patterns from their early years into the later stages of life. In the view of Heinz Kohut, the founder of self-psychology, the self develops out of interaction with certain key nurturing figures in the caretaking environment that he terms "selfobjects"—the significant people who represent the object world (Fonagy, 2001). These selfobjects do not simply gratify the infant's biological needs and desires, but provide key functions that strengthen and support the development of a more realistic and positive sense of the self in the growing child. These selfobject functions may comfort, control tension, and help maintain stability of the self-system (Greenberg & Mitchell, 1983). As the infant matures, he or she internalizes these functions as a way to strengthen his/her own growing sense of self and regulate his/her self-esteem. A simple example would be the way in which a person learns to cope with disappointment and loss at an early age.

Kohut, like Fairbairn before him, departed from the classical drive model and instead focused on the development of the self—a structure contained in the ego (Kohut, 1977). Kohut's developmental model is predicated on the idea that "the individual is born with an innate sense of self, which is the central organizing and motivating force in the personality but also requires an empathic and responsive selfobject environment in order of unfold optimally" (Goldstein, 2001, p. 42).

Kohut emphasized the importance of two distinct object functions in his relational configuration:

1 *Mirroring* takes place in a nurturing context in which the infant can begin to feel more known, more real, and more internally substantial. The maternal figure is responsive to the infant and reflects back enthusiasm, approval, and praise that reinforce the infant's spontaneously arising healthy narcissism. For example, the caretaker can respond with a loving smile, a proud gaze, or a soothing touch.
2 *Idealizing*, in which the infant needs to form an idealized image of at least one parent and experience a sense of merger with this idealized selfobject. By feeling an essential likeness with the much-admired, omnipotent parent, the immature self feels stronger and more powerful (Mitchell & Black, 1995).

In the context of these two functions, the child experiences the mother's pride or disinterest as the acceptance or rejection of his or her active self. It is normal and necessary for a child to seek confirming, approving responses from a mother figure; our pursuit of recognition and attention offsets some of the loneliness and desire for closeness we feel throughout life. Like Sullivan, Kohut believes that individuals require a milieu of empathically responding selfobjects throughout their lives to gain recognition and attention. If we do not experience warmth and closeness, it is difficult to remain an active agent in any aspect of life.

Kohut assumes that most individuals are born into a responsive human milieu. However, this is not always true, and relatedness with others, a condition necessary for psychological survival, cannot be taken for granted. If parents' needs are unmet, it is harder for them to be appropriately responsive to the child (Rowe & Mac Isaac, 1991). This suggests that in order to help the child, the social worker must help the parent to repair early deprivations or trauma.

Kohut's psychology of the self has profound implications for the client–worker relationship in that he emphasizes empathic sensitivity to the client's subjective experience and recognition of the need for life-long selfobjects. This focus raises the question of whether the worker can function as a positive selfobject for individuals who lack a stable sense of self and identity, and are vulnerable to sudden losses of self-esteem. Alternatively, can the clinician help the client seek new selfobject functions in the present environment, in the form of nurturing figures or caregivers, to compensate for earlier deficits?

Kohut's belief that personality disorders can be attributed to early deficits in selfobject introjections suggests that the clinician may compensate for less than adequate early relationships—at least to some degree—by creating an empathic, accepting environment where the worker is tuned into the client's needs and wants (Mitchell, 1988). Furthermore, Kohut's work offers the possibility that a more positive self-concept can be formed through favorable interactions with sensitive, caring, and validating persons in the environment. Basing clinical work on the understanding that the relationship between client and worker permits new object relations to form thus reinforces the value social work has placed on the helping relationship.

In summary, the schools of self-psychology, object relations, and interpersonal theory furthered relational thinking by proposing the following:

- While the individual is born with an innate sense of self, the child needs a responsive and empathic environment (caregivers) to achieve a coherent sense of self.
- Relationships are at the center of human experience.
- Individuals need close relationships to perform certain empathic responses.
- Individuals need relational opportunities to develop optimally across the life cycle (Goldstein et al., 2009).

Intersubjectivity theory

Object relations theory serves as a bridge to the intersubjective approach to clinical practice. According to Robert Stolorow and his colleagues, George Atwood and Bernard Brandschaft, a person's primary experience of self, self-esteem, and personality has its origins in the degree to which mutual regulation exists in the subjective world of the child–primary caretaker system. This intersubjective world includes shared ideas, emotions, impressions; it places the psyche in the realm of interacting human systems. An important indicator of well-being is the subjective reality of how the client experiences relationships and events. Stolorow believed that the internalization of infant–caregiver patterns result in mental structures that organize the child's subjective experience and have an influence on later interactions with others (Stolorow et al., 1994).

Jessica Benjamin (1988), a feminist thinker and psychoanalyst, articulates an intersubjective view. Benjamin maintains that the individual grows in and through the relationship to other subjects. She goes further than other intersubjective theorists in her attempt to place the relational nature of human experience in a gendered specific social context. She suggests that gender differences, which underlie false polarities in our society, such as assertiveness and independence (associated with male socialization) and submissiveness and dependence (associated with female socialization), create tension between the need for autonomy and the need for connection in individuals. As she sees it, the need for mutual recognition—the necessity of recognizing as well as being recognized by others—serves as an equalizer and a unifying concept for such dualisms. Benjamin questions the tendency in psychoanalytic thinking to polarize the child as "subject" and the mother as "object." She reconceptualizes the psychic world as "a subject meeting another subject" (1988, p. 20).

Benjamin rejects the notion of traditional object relations theorists that mother and infant are merged at birth. Instead, she develops a feminist orientation, asserting that the self develops its structure in the presence of a shifting balance of connection and differentiation. Self-representations characterized by clear but flexible boundaries and appreciation of difference from important others exist alongside self-representations in which self and other overlap.

Relational–cultural theory

The founders of relational–cultural theory credit Robert Stolorow and colleagues as having a major influence on their theory. The relational–cultural school of thought is a relatively new approach to practice developed by a group of female clinicians and scholars at the Stone Center at Wellesley College in the 1970s. This group of women came together to develop a relational model of practice that emphasized the centrality of connection in women's lives. This theoretical framework is compatible with the core practice principles and values of direct social work practice and provides a contextual view of self that is consistent with both the person-in-situation, cultural competency, and the ecological systems perspective.

While most developmental theories devised by men generally emphasize the growth of an autonomous, individuated self, women's experience, in large measure, contradicts such theory. According to Miller and Stiver (1997), women's sense of self is, to a great degree, organized around being able to make and then maintain affiliation and relationship. In other words, psychological growth and development takes place in and through increasingly complex relationships over the life cycle.

Traditional theories of human growth and development have usually relied on research using male subjects conditioned by the male experience in a Western industrialized society (Erikson, 1950; Levinson, 1978; Kohlberg, 1981). Rooted in cultural standards and expectations which value the ideals of competition, individual mastery, and independence, mature psychological development was expected to evolve out of a dyadic relationship with the primary caretaker through increasing levels of separation and individuation (Erikson, 1968; Mahler et al., 1975). Applying these principles of male development to women made them seem deficient rather than merely different.

Carol Gilligan

Carol Gilligan (1982) is one of the first feminist theorists to note that the discrepancy between women's experience and the prevailing theories of human development was generally considered to represent a problem in female development. According to Gilligan, what is missing from those theories is the idea that the development of the self and morality takes place within relationships and is embedded in a relational context which changes over time. In essence, she constructed a theory of the different ways women think about rights and responsibilities.

In her seminal book *In a Different Voice*, Gilligan (1982) rejects Lawrence Kohlberg's stage theory of moral development to make her argument that women fare less well than men in traditional theories of psychological and moral development. Kohlberg's theory, which centers on the development of what he calls the "justice" perspective, attributes a higher level of maturity to individuals who make moral decisions based on their own sense of what they believe is right and true, independently of others (Kohlberg, 1981). Gilligan argued that this approach does not accurately reflect women's development and experiences across the life cycle—experiences that socialize women to make decisions with their personal interest and concern for others in mind. Her attempt to correct the male bias in Kohlberg's theory gave impetus to the development of her relational ethics of responsibility and care.

Gilligan's relational theory of responsibility and care represents an attempt to re-conceptualize the relationship between judgment and action, thought and experience, concepts of self and morality, and experiences of conflict and choice. She describes women as tending to hear a "different voice" than men when thinking through personal and moral decisions. After extensive empirical observations of different ways in which women think about rights and responsibilities, Gilligan concluded that women's experiences and perspectives, and their overriding concern with relationships and responsibilities, had a major effect on their decision-making processes in a myriad of ways. For example, Gilligan's classic abortion decision study of 30 women of diverse ethnic backgrounds revealed that their decision about whether or not to have an abortion was based on what was in the best interest of the unborn baby; most of the women ultimately made a decision based on their sense of their ability to care for and protect the other (Gilligan, 1982).

Based on the abortion decision study and other empirical observations, Gilligan concluded that women's experiences, and their concern with relationships and responsibilities, had a major effect on their decision-making processes. She found that girls and women are more likely to equate morality with helping and pleasing others than with the inclination, characteristic of many of the males in Kohlberg's study, to make decisions and moral judgments in terms of an abstract principle of justice. Women's experiences revealed that they learn about the world in relation to others, basing their decisions on a sense of care balanced by intellectual reasoning (Gilligan, 1982).

Nancy Chodorow

Like Gilligan, feminist sociologist and psychoanalyst Nancy Chodorow (1978) highlighted the difference between developmental pathways for boys and girls based on gender-specific social structures and cultural arrangements. Specifically, she was concerned with disparities in male–female participation in child rearing. Since the majority of primary caregivers for young children in our society are women, it is natural that boys and girls will be affected differently in their personality formation and gender identity development, beginning as early as the pre-Oedipal stage.

However, Chodorow suggests that "gender difference is not absolute ... and the experience of difference is socially and psychologically created" (1990, p. 42). Using object relations and psychoanalytic theory, Chodorow describes how girls internalize aspects of mothering—care, empathy, and softness, for example—in their identification with their same-sex parent. These traits are re-enacted with their own children and are eventually reproduced psychologically and sociologically across generations.

According to Chodorow, early self-representations characterized by clear but flexible boundaries cohere around specific interactions with the early nurturing figure(s) and contribute to the development of a "relational self" in women. Girls continue to identify with their mothers who are expected to provide the nurturing and relational context of the early years; they internalize the qualities that are crucial to the ability to achieve interpersonal connectedness. In their search for a strong masculine identity in the early years of life, boys reject those "soft" qualities associated with a nurturing maternal figure. Thus, ego boundaries become more rigid in boys than girls in an effort to protect and secure their masculine identity (Chodorow, 1978).

While Chodorow recognized that qualities of the mother–daughter relationship vary, and that generations change with regard to parental responsibility, she believed that the reproduction of feminine traits associated with the mother–daughter relationship is firmly embedded in the majority culture (Chodorow, 1994).

As time moves on, it has becomes clear that the relational/cultural framework has relevance for males as well as females. Data reveal that, more so than in the past, men are in the position of raising children and are seeking new definitions of what it means to be a man and a parent. Many modern fathers believe in the importance of connection with their children and of providing a positive relational context for growth and development for both themselves and their children (Watson-Phillips, 2006).

Stephen Bergman (1991) argues that, like women, men also desire connection. However, unlike women, male socialization encourages a sense of self as separate from the other. In order to become a "man," the young boy is supposed to relinquish his intimate relationship with his mother in order to develop an identity that is based on the Western paradigm of 'being your own man.'

Stone Center for Research and Developmental Studies

Building on relational concepts from psychology and the work of Benjamin, Gilligan, and Chodorow, the founding leaders from the Stone Center for Research and Developmental Studies at Wellesley College, Jean Baker Miller, Alexandra Kaplan, Judith Jordan, Irene Stiver, and Janet Surrey (Jordan et al., 1991a) noted the failure of traditional psychologists and developmental theorists to fully appreciate the relational nature of women's sense of themselves. Stone Center scholars and clinicians proposed an interactive sense of self as a paradigm for the study of all self-in-environment experience. In essence, the common organizing principle in this approach to clinical work is that all growth occurs "in connection," and that all people desire connection and growth-fostering relationships which are created by mutual empathy and mutual empowerment (Jordan & Hartling, 2002).

The Stone Center model views connections, disconnections, and re-connections in relationships as core developmental processes. Originally termed self-in-relation theory by Jean Baker Miller (Jordan et al., 1991b) the model emphasizes the fact that for women, the self is organized, developed, and maintained in the context of important relationships throughout life (Surrey, 1991c). It posits that optimally: (1) we grow in, through, and toward relationship; (2) for women, especially, connection with others is central to psychological well-being; and (3) movement toward relational mutuality can occur throughout life, through mutual empathy and responsiveness (Jordan, 1997a; Kaplan, 1991b; Miller & Stiver, 1997; Spencer, 2000).

In her ground-breaking book *Toward a New Psychology of Women* (1976), Jean Baker Miller laid the foundation for a female-centered relational perspective on practice which she called "self-in-relation" theory. She argued that power inequality in male and female gender roles relegated females to a subordinate position vis-à-vis males in this society, and suggested that, to the extent to which mutually enhancing interactions are unlikely in situations of unequal power, growth may require acknowledging difference and openly engaging in conflict.

Miller further proposed that the role, function, and social situation of women in a male-dominated society—involving the social structuring of gendered relationships—is intrinsically connected to understanding the development of mind, identity, and self. She argued that women develop a sense of self in a context of attachment and affiliation with others, while most men build their identity through increasing levels of autonomy and separation. Thus, the female sense of self becomes organized, to a considerable extent, around being able to make and then maintain relationships. For example, it is much more likely that a female suffering from depression has experienced the loss of affiliation with others, while a man is more likely be depressed due to the loss of a job or some other status symbol that reflects society's affirmation of his manhood.

Jean Baker Miller (1991a) challenged traditional developmental theorists, such as Erik Erikson and Margaret Mahler, who viewed ego development as a process of separating oneself out from the matrix of a "fused" existence with another. Instead, she suggested that from the moment of birth, the development of an internal representation of self takes place in active interchange with other selves—what she calls "being in relationship." Miller proposed that the infant begins to be and act like the main caregiver, identifying not only with the caregiver as "some static figure described only by gender, but with what the person is actually doing" (1991a, p. 31). Thus, the infant begins to develop an internal differentiated representation of him or herself within close connection to another within the first few months of life: "The child experiences a sense of comfort only as the other is also comfortable, or, a little more accurately, as they are both engaged in an emotional relationship that is moving toward greater well-being" (Miller, 1991a, p. 3).

This movement toward mutuality is central to successful coping and healthy development. As Judith Jordan (1991d, p. 1) eloquently states: "Movement toward mutuality lies at the heart of relational development. Rather than viewing people as primarily motivated by a need for self-sufficiency and personal gratification, a relational perspective acknowledges our deep need to establish connections with other people."

In relationships characterized by mutuality, individuals relate to one another based on an interest in each other as whole, complex persons and with an awareness of the other's subjective experience. In such an exchange, one both affects the other and is affected by the other; one extends oneself out to the other and is also receptive to the impact of the other (Jordan, 1991b).

The emphasis on mutuality proposes a major paradigm shift in Western psychology from a psychology of the separate self to a psychology of relational being. Jordan (1997a) traces several biases in the traditional view of the self; one such bias being the emphasis on the self as a bounded, discrete, entity, that has influenced psychoanalytic theory in the Western industrialized world. She asserts that, to gain authority, psychology as a discipline has modeled itself on the "hard" sciences (such as physics) rather than as an extension of a humanistic tradition associated with female sensibilities. She writes: "Newtonian physics posited discrete, separate entities existing in space and acting on each other in predictable and measureable ways. This easily led to a study of the self as a comparably bounded and contained 'molecular entity'" (Jordan, 1997a, p. 10).

According to Jordan, the belief in a "separate self" acts as a barrier to a shared understanding of the psychological state of others, making fluid, reciprocal interchanges between people difficult. The concept of empathy—the dynamic cognitive process of joining with and understanding another's subjective experience—is central to Jordan's intention of altering the traditional boundaries between subject and object and promoting an inter-subjective notion of relationship (Jordan, 1991a).

The relational–cultural approach emphasizes the nature and quality of connectedness to others. According to Janet Surrey (1991c), early self-representations characterized by clear but flexible boundaries cohere around specific interactions with the primary nurturing figure and contribute to the development of a "relational self" in women. Contrary to traditional psychological theory that suggests aspects of the self unfolding along a developmental line of increasing autonomy, separation, and independence, Surrey (1991c) argues that the self develops its structure in the presence of a finely tuned, shifting balance of connection and differentiation with significant others. In other words, she shifts the emphasis from separation and individuation to relationship with differentiation as a goal for healthy functioning. This model might be expressed as: *Rather than separate completely from you, I am going to define who I am in relation to you. Interaction with you allows me to get a better sense of myself than I could get on my own, so I'm going to stay connected to you.* Thus relational theory affords the opportunity to appreciate the relational nature of women's sense of self, rather than judging their identity formation as deficient or lacking in some fundamental way.

In essence, the common organizing principle in this approach to clinical social work is the capacity for, and continuity of, relationships in women's and men's ordinary life experiences. For social work practice, the pathway toward development of a healthy sense of self includes helping the client reach increasing levels of choice, complexity, mutuality, and satisfaction in his/her constellation of relationships.

In the mid to late 1980s, using Baker Miller's work as a springboard, theoreticians and clinicians at the Stone Center for Developmental Services and Studies at Wellesley College expanded on the self-in-relation perspective and came to refer to it as the "relational–cultural" model in order to emphasize the fact that psycho-social development takes place in and through increasingly complex cultural, social, and relational contexts (Miller & Stiver, 1997). The relational–cultural approach emphasizes the impact of variables such as gender, class, ethnicity, and sexual preference—in fact the entire context in which societies are organized—on the experiences of everyday relationships as well as levels of connectedness in communities and society as a whole.

A relational–cultural paradigm for clinical practice creates a framework for examining the interaction between cultural norms and social systems at different levels: family, organization, community, etc. Cultural and social forces have a great impact on how individuals value themselves, the resources available to them, and the nature of their relationships with others. Along with cultural role expectations, politics, social privilege, as well as economic and class restrictions, affect people's level of psycho-social functioning. An awareness of different ethnic groups, their degrees of marginalization, and their family norms and values must be factored into the knowledge and skill of the clinician working with a diverse clientele.

The acceptance of the other's differentness in a relationship can provide a powerful sense of validation for both people. According to Jordan, "Growth occurs because I stretch to match or understand your experiences, something new is acknowledged and grows in me" (1986, p. 3). The relational–cultural school advances an understanding of the emotional, social, moral, and cognitive development of girls and women in its particular sensitivity to the life experiences of females within diverse cultural contexts.

The relational/cultural model is sometimes referred to in this book as the feminist relational paradigm because it embraces a political and economic analysis of patriarchy. Many women experience a sense of oppression as a result of having accepted and internalized the cultural devaluation of their experiences and the perceived limitations in their development. By clarifying the cultural norms surrounding the notions of "masculinity" and "femininity" in our society, the practitioner can raise the consciousness of both male and female clients.

Research and relational inventories

In recent years, psychologists have begun to develop measurement tools based on relational theory for evaluation and assessment purposes (Frey, 2013). Two tools are noteworthy. In 1992, Genero, Miller, and Surrey developed the Mutual Psychological Development Questionnaire, a 22-item self-report scale that measures perceived mutuality in close relationships (see Appendix A). Based on the relational framework of Miller and Surrey, Genero et al. identified six key elements of mutual interaction— empathy, engagement, authenticity, empowerment, zest, and diversity. Genero and her associates then operationalized these concepts as follows:

1   Empathy: The process by which one person experiences the feelings and thoughts of another and simultaneously knows her/his own different feelings and thoughts (e.g. pick up on my feelings).
2   Engagement: The focusing on one another in a meaningful way (e.g. show an interest).
3   Authenticity: The process of coming closer to knowing and sharing one's experience with another. Seeing and recognizing the other for who she/he is and being seen and recognized for who one is (e.g. share similar experiences; avoid being honest; keep feelings inside).
4   Empowerment: The capacity for action that emerges from connection within a relationship. To participate in an interaction in such a way that one simultaneously enhances one's own capacity to act as well as the other's (e.g. express an opinion clearly).
5   Zest: Feelings of vitality, aliveness, energy, enjoyment, and gusto (e.g. see the humor in things).
6   Diversity: The process of openly expressing and receiving different perspectives, opinion, and feelings (e.g. respect my point of view).

Preliminary findings show that the Mutual Psychological Development Questionnaire (MPDQ) may be helpful as a research instrument for future clinical applications.

The Relational Health Indices (RHI) developed by Liang et al. (1998) are based on the relational–cultural theory of Jordan et al. (1991a). It is an exploratory study in which four dimensions of growth fostering relationships were included in a questionnaire and administered to 450 students in an all-women's liberal arts college: engagement/empathy; empowerment/zest; authenticity; and difference/conflict. The validity of these measures tested positively along the dimensions of peer, community, and mentoring relationships and was published as *Relational Health Indices: An Exploratory Study* (see Appendix B of this book).

This study of relational health of growth-fostering relationships represents an exciting direction for future research and supports the beneficial qualities of relationships that (1) are mutual and respectful, (2) can facilitate emotional resiliency and coping strategies, and (3) provide motivation for reaching out for additional social supports.

At about the same time, D. Griffin and K. Bartholomew published their Relationship Scales Questionnaire (RSQ), designed as a continuous measure of adult attachment (1994). These scales reflect degrees of security, fearfulness, preoccupation, and dismissing that can be used to rate the development of these relational factors over time. The questionnaire consisted of 30 items in which participants were asked to rate themselves on a five-point scale. Items were general statements about ease of relationships; for example, "I find it difficult to depend on other people." The RSQ was not designed nor intended to be used as a categorical measure of attachment. Rather, researchers examined whether attachment styles had an effect on interaction anxiety in college freshmen.

Neurological theory

Emerging neuroscience information has confirmed that our emotions and behavior affect our brain chemistry and that alterations in brain chemistry affect our emotions and behavior. Neuroscience is the study of the brain's neurons, or nerve cells that send and receive electro-chemical signals to and from the brain and nervous system. Neuroscience is sometimes used interchangeably with neurobiology which studies the organizational structure of nerve cells, the actual neuronal networks that process information and regulate behavior. Neuropsychology, a subset of neuroscience, studies the structure and function of the brain as it relates to psychological processes and behaviors (Siegel, 2012).

At the heart of brain studies is the interconnection between the physical and psychological aspects of our functioning. Twenty-five years ago the general consensus among neuroscientists was that the adult brain was considered a static organ and that its regenerative capacities came to an end once adulthood was reached. However, we now know that:

- The brain has the capacity to create new individual neurons (neurogenesis).
- The brain generates new synaptic networks and/or modifies existing ones (neuroplasticity).
- Interaction between neurons is the fuel that sparks the fires of both neurogenesis and neuroplasticity.

Neuroscience and relational–cultural theory

In his book *The Neuroscience of Human Relationships*, Cozolino (2006) explores the ways in which interpersonal interactions shape the structure of not only our own brains, but the brains of each other, an idea echoed by Siegel when he states "that human connections create neural connection" (2012, p. 3). According to Cozolino and Siegel, our brains are unable to survive without relational experience, indicating that perhaps the time has come to finally forego the nature versus nurture debate in favor of the research data indicating that we are neurologically wired for connection. The findings of interpersonal neurobiology suggest that the function and structure of the brain is continually being shaped by our emotional relationships.

The relational nature of brain development reflects the view of relational–cultural theory which focuses on relationship as a model of human growth and a primary path to maturity. Cozolino has developed the social brain theory of human development, a model in which all brains need other brains for mutually stimulating interactions; otherwise, they wither and die. As a social organ that is built through experience, Cozolino believes that the brain is fundamentally shaped through our relationships with other people (i.e. other brains). No longer is adulthood measured by the degree to which we are autonomous and separate from others. Instead, it is based on our relational experiences, on our bonds and affinities with others (Cozolino, 2006).

Through Cozolino's work we are learning that connections and disconnections not only occur at a personal and societal level, but at a biological level as well. While the process of neuroplaticity can form new connections in our brains at incredible speeds, in order for our neural circuitry to redesign itself it must be prompted by our relational experience. The familiar axiom "neurons that fire together, wire together" also works in reverse: neurons that do not regularly fire together separate from one another and form autonomous circuits (Siegel, 2012, p. 3).

Interpersonal neurobiology and social brain theory may one day lead us toward the recognition that men and women are more alike than different, for both male and female brains use the experience of connection and disconnection as the primary means for structuring and restructuring neuropathways. Perhaps the qualities of relationship that foster healthy brain growth in women will ultimately prove to be the same qualities that foster healthy brain growth in men, raising a new set of questions surrounding the different psychological tool-kits each gender has developed in order to function within dominant hierarchies. What would it mean to discover that connection, not separation, is the guiding principle of growth for both men and women?

Research data reveal that human beings are continuously formed within the context of relational experience which in turn continuously alters brain development. If this is the case, than healing interaction can stimulate changes that help people release suffering and grow in positive ways. According to Stone Center psychiatrist Dr. Amy Banks, psychotherapy needs to recognize that relationships extend beyond abstract psychodynamic concepts. They are actual neuronal, structural configurations that illustrate relational connections and disconnections. Honoring emotional injuries (and their accompanying disconnections) supports the client's development of a new relational template built upon respect, patience, and understanding, and the brain responds in kind by constructing new neuropathways that match the new relational qualities (Banks, 2010).

Current therapeutic questions under investigation include: How do therapists and educators stimulate the brain's neuroplastic processes to create change and create well-being? What are the processes through which relationship creates mental illness or mental health? Neuroscience has allowed us to make a quantum leap in our understanding of the human condition, and will continue to provide the backdrop for therapeutic considerations as we move forward.

3   The client–worker relationship

This chapter focuses on the use of feminist relational concepts in the client–worker relationship. Since social work's mission involves change, this would include using the professional relationship in ways that move clients out of their isolation, out of destructive relationships, and into connections that are more growth producing. Not only are social workers uniquely positioned to create the kinds of relationship that enhance self-esteem and mobilize client strengths, but they can also observe and assess clients' relationships with other social systems, such as school personnel, work colleagues, neighbors, and extended family.

There are many different types of relationships in individuals' lives, the client–worker being just one prototype of what a relationship can be. Guided by the Stone Center Works in Progress series, the relational–cultural model requires the worker to focus attention on the client's relational processes, the structural components of relationships, and the implications of chronic disconnection. As suggested by Nancy Chodorow (1978), an inner sense of connection to others is a central organizing feature in women's development. Social and cultural mores have made it easier for females to seek out relationships and to stay connected longer than males. However, the internalized gendered world is not fixed, and the desire for connection can cut across gender lines, particularly in today's changing society.

A feminist relational viewpoint places emphasis on relational yearnings as normative, not only connected to unresolved residues of childhood, as some psychodynamic theorists have argued (Greenberg & Mitchell, 1983). Since we all replay significant relational dynamics, the potential power in the therapeutic relationship lies in the opportunity to provide the client with a reparative experience. This relationship can then serve as a model for other relationships—ones in which the client can both reshape internal negative images resulting from past hurt, and reconstruct other relationships in more positive ways. This desire for relationship, considered to be a life-long motivating force that drives feeling, thought, and action, reinforces the importance social workers have given to a dynamic systems approach, in which the emphasis is on interaction. Beebe and Lachmann (2002) documented infants as young as three months adjusting their behavior to their mothers' movements, supporting the notion of interaction as continuous and mutually constructed, a reciprocal form of attunement people engage in throughout life.

The therapeutic goal is to create a deeper, more meaningful sense of connection between worker and client and between client and others. An authentic and responsive relational context, characterized by mutuality, reciprocity, and intersubjectivity, has the potential to enhance clients' capacity to cope under adverse circumstances and to promote adaptation under normative ones. The energy of the client–worker relationship can become the fuel for decision making that enhances clients' ability to take action. Simply put, social workers are change agents, and relationships marked by mutuality can facilitate the helping process. Social workers can also be role models who help people learn how to relate to others in healthier ways. Just as mothers and fathers are not born knowing how to parent but must learn these skills through practice, so people learn how to relate to others through modeling, identification, and education.

Exploring all of the client's relationships—present *and* past—may prove highly significant in understanding them. For example, a father who abandoned his child years ago and is absent in the child's day-to-day life may be *the* most important variable to consider when working with that child and his or her family. Yet the inexperienced social worker may overlook this.

The social work relationship: traditional approaches, contemporary trends

While relationship has been traditionally defined as the basic condition in which two or more people with some common interest connect, the advent of globalization and increased immigration make it increasingly important for social workers to relate to clients with greater cultural sensitivity. Concepts such as dependency, use of self, transference–countertransference, and boundaries as traditionally interpreted may no longer fit the diverse populations with whom we work.

The client–worker relationship

The role of the client–worker relationship has long occupied a prominent position in direct social work practice, particularly in casework, which dominated the field from the 1920s through the 1960s. Virginia Robinson (1930) credited the client–worker relationship with the ability to provide internal support needed to bolster ego functions and to redress imbalances when coping with stress and facing challenges. Later, Helen Harris Perlman (1979) pointed out that the essence of what social workers do takes place in the interchange between ourselves and other people, and suggested that relationships have the potential to sustain us throughout life, affirming our sense of identity as well as a sense of oneness with others. These far-reaching therapeutic powers invested in the social work relationship discussed earlier in our history still holds true today.

Much of the professional literature continues to maintain that a healthy client–worker relationship infuses the helping process with energy and hope and becomes a medium through which to mobilize clients' strengths. Jeanne Marsh (2005) observes that "social workers know that the connection between the worker and the client is the most powerful tool available to social workers, regardless of the treatment approach or modality they may be using" (p. 195). Relationships are the essence of our existence and continually influence and define who we are, how we feel, what we do, and the ways we live our lives.

According to Woods and Hollis (1999), the social work relationship can be a model for handling problems that arise with other people in our clients' lives. The client has the opportunity to identify with and incorporate the worker's strengths in learning how to deal more effectively with difficult situations. While social work practitioners have always been concerned with the client–worker relationship, the focus has traditionally been on coping with problems. In the feminist relational approach, however, the emphasis shifts from merely coping, to growth and empowerment.

Most discussions of the professional relationship have revolved mainly around a description of essential worker characteristics that have been proven effective in establishing and sustaining a productive working relationship. Compton et al. (2005) summarize these characteristics by stating that the social worker:

- evidences warmth;
- displays empathy;
- shows acceptance;
- is concerned;
- is genuine and congruent;
- shows commitment and obligation; and
- uses authority and power appropriately.

Felix Biestek (1957) considered the relationship between worker and client to be "the channel of the entire casework process; through it flows the skills in intervention, study, diagnosis and treatment" (p. 4). He identified seven key features in the social work relationship reflecting professional values that promote growth and change and which continue to guide social work practice today: (1) individualization; (2) purposeful expression of feeling; (3) controlled emotional involvement; (4) acceptance; (5) non-judgmental attitude; (6) client self-determination; and (7) confidentiality.

While Biestek made an important contribution to practice, he does not identify mutuality as one of the key features in the client–worker relationship. The feminist relational approach places emphasis on the therapeutic milieu characterized by a sense of mutuality—a two-way interactive connection. It implicates the full range of emotions and thoughts that naturally flow between two or more persons. Thus, the client–worker dyad needs to be looked at as a behavioral system that functions in a reciprocal manner within a particular social and cultural milieu. This notion of mutuality is a key feature in the feminist relational approach and sets it apart from more traditional social work perspectives.

Mutuality

Over the past decade, the Stone Center for Research and Clinical Studies has highlighted mutuality as a central component of a healthy relationship. The underlying assumption rests on the concept that mutual need and mutual aid are implicit in every society where interdependence ultimately leads to growth rather than isolation (Shulman, 2006). The notion of mutuality, implicit in the philosophy of a feminist relational approach, is often missing in the social work literature.

According to Stone Center pioneer Judith Jordan (1991c), the mutual exchange with a client is a setting in which "one is affecting the others and is being affected by the other; one that extends oneself out to the other and is also receptive to the impact of the other" (p. 82). Simply stated, mutuality is the idea of reciprocity in relationship. Inherent in this approach is (1) an appreciation of the other as a unique, whole person; (2) an interest in and a cognitive awareness of the other's subjective state (who the other is, what he or she thinks and feels); (3) an ability to reveal one's own inner states to another; (4) a capacity to acknowledge one's own needs without manipulating the other; (5) a valuing of the process of enhancing the other's growth; and (6) a pattern of interaction in which both people are open to change.

Mutuality does not mean that each person in the relationship has equal power. Nor does mutuality imply an experience of sameness with the other. Appreciating differences while maintaining connection in a mutual exchange can be growth enhancing if there is sufficient respect, an understanding of the other's experience, an ongoing interest in their inner world, and the willingness to allow oneself to be affected by it (Jordan, 1991c). While the movement toward mutuality requires attunement to the client's needs, it is not necessarily direct, immediate, or even continuous; it may be prone to fits and starts. The social worker can employ the following means in order to encourage the reciprocal impact of the worker and client system (Jordan et al., 1991):

- Disclose personal information as appropriate.
- Let the client know what you have learned from them.
- Consider that the client has the most expertise on his or her problem.
- Accept and validate the client's experiences, feelings, thoughts, and perceptions about you as a professional helper.
- Express care and concern about the client.

First and foremost, the client–worker relationship is seen as a partnership. In a non-dichotomous model, growth comes from the client's ability to become increasingly active within the relationship, eventually acting upon the environment with greater assertion (Kaplan, 1988). In many ways, technique is secondary to the worker's attitude embodied in these qualities:

- mutual respect;
- emotional availability;
- relational authenticity;
- relational awareness;
- responsiveness and presence;
- openness to influence.

The case of Linda, a 30-year-old, second-generation Dominican young woman, illustrates the impact of mutuality on the client–worker relationship. Linda told me that she suffers from depression, and has always had a difficult time asserting herself with others. Subsequent to her divorce one year ago, she related that she was feeling isolated and lonely, and that it was hard for her to reach out to others. I had worked with Linda for about two months when she shared that she was having an affair with a married man at work. This relationship was basically the only gratifying one she had outside of her relationship with me. While Linda gave to others easily, she could not assert her own needs in return; hence, her relationships lacked mutuality.

Christmas and New Year were fast approaching and Linda was feeling particularly alone since her "boyfriend" would be with his wife. She dared not tell her parents or siblings about this relationship for fear of their judgment of her. They are religious, church-going people, who would view Linda's behavior as sinful. Her mother's strong tie to her Hispanic culture and Linda's acculturation into the Anglo culture only widened the gap between them. Her mother does not speak much English, nor does her world extend beyond where she lives and works. The literature indicates that close relationships between young Hispanic females and their mothers, when there is mutuality, understanding, and empathy, are protective factors that can help young Latina women to negotiate the demands of both mainstream and Hispanic cultures. A close mother–daughter relationship has been correlated with higher levels of self-esteem and lower levels of depression (Genero et al., 1992). These findings are echoed in Linda's case.

I knew from previous sessions with Linda that when she becomes "down on herself," she retreats from others. I shared with Linda that her withdrawal and self-imposed isolation concerned me, given a previous suicide attempt she had made, and especially since the holidays are generally the worst times for many people. At the moment I said these words to her I felt Linda moving away from me.

In the past Linda had been teased and ridiculed by peers in school, her former mother-in-law, and her former husband because of her depression and learning problems. Repeated disconnections have been a part of Linda's life and she automatically avoids or retreats from others when she does not want to talk about something painful or when she feels uncomfortable. Linda lowered her head, became reticent, and moved her chair back. I felt disconnected from her and any attempt I made to empathize or reach out seemed useless. I said that I felt she was distancing herself from me as she does with others in her life when she is upset. I reminded her that I cared about her, and felt sad that she was feeling so alone—I wanted to help her, not hurt her.

Since Linda could not rely on her mother for a sense of connectedness, our relationship took on heightened significance. I let her know that I wanted to be there for her, and I felt frustrated and helpless that she had withdrawn from me emotionally. I imagined that she might also feel the same frustration and helplessness. I asked, "Are you beginning to give up on yourself again?" I let her know that in the past I too had withdrawn from others when I was in emotional pain, or when I felt "down on myself," and those were the times when I needed other people the most. At those words, Linda started to cry. Her tears provided a way for her to express the painful well of emptiness that kept her so removed from others.

The reciprocal exchange that takes place in the client–worker relationship is made possible by the capacity of each participant for mutuality. As noted earlier, researchers have presented evidence that from birth, infants can express their intentions and needs to their caregiver, which results in a process of mutual regulation (Stern, 1985). Each member's actions are the complement of the partner; one person performs the action, the other receives it. The reciprocal low of energy invested in the client–worker relationship sets the change process in motion. More recent research (Tronick & Weinberg, 1997, p. 56) suggests that patterns of differentiation of self and other exist almost from birth:

> Exchanges with interactive partners which are well regulated generate positive affect, while mismatched exchanges produce negative affect. The expression of these affective states in turn communicates to the interactive partner to continue what he or she is doing or to change interactive behaviors.

Mutuality rarely happens from the onset. Relationships evolve, change, and grow over time within multi-dimensional relational and cultural contexts. Helping clients connect with their full range of reactions, including the impact made on them by the social worker, enriches the dynamics of the interaction. Conversely, when social workers are able to connect with the impact clients have made on them, a truly relational experience is created.

In my relationship with Linda, I found it helpful to understand that because of past traumas and repeated disconnections, sometimes, those who yearn for connection the most hide parts of themselves from others as well as from themselves. Miller and Stiver (1995) call this phenomenon the paradox of connection. The knowledgeable clinician, using mutually empathic skills, is aware of both sides of the dilemma: the desire on one side for secure attachment, and the fear of continued rejection or harm on the other. Children and adults alike use various strategies to either retreat into their private worlds or to act out aggressively to keep people away as a means of self-protection.

Worker's use of self

The practice of feminist relational social work challenges professionals to critically reflect on the ways in which they use themselves in the helping relationship. The use of self is an ambiguous concept, and arguably one that has never been fully elaborated upon in the social work literature. Perhaps if we start by examining the use of self in the feminist relational approach we can better understand how social work can make use of this fundamental idea. In the relational cultural approach, the use of self is bound up with notions of mutuality, authenticity, boundaries, self-disclosure, transference and countertransference issues, all of which are discussed in this chapter. Although these concepts overlap in practice, they are discussed separately for the purpose of clarification.

Although there may not be consensus on exactly what is meant by the use of self, clearly the worker's own unique self permeates his or her practice. Components of the worker's self include personality, culture, appearance, age, ethnicity, gender, and sexual orientation. Entering into another person's space requires sensitivity, knowledge, patience, compassion, skill, and keen self-awareness. All of these aspects of the self intersect and produce more than the sum of each part, encompassing a totally different and more elaborate cultural medium in which relational dynamics take place (Germain & Gitterman, 1996).

According to Jordan (1991c), in everyday life, "the other person is not there merely to take care of one's needs, to become a vessel for one's projections or transferences, or to be an object of discharge of instinctual impulses" (p. 82). By extension, when the client can see more than "just another social worker" in front of them, and can relate to the practitioner as a whole and separate individual, there is the potential for the client to become more invested in the helping process. If clients can then transfer this increased relational capacity to others in their lives, they become more effective in negotiating their environment and in forming healthier connections with others.

A brief example will illustrate this. After I had worked with Nina for three years, she missed a session and did not call. I phoned to see what had happened and left a message. She did not call back until the following week. When we explored the meaning of her missed session, Nina herself connected her behavior with her tendency to avoid what she anticipated might be difficult; she wanted to terminate but did not know how to bring it up. I asked her how she thought I felt when she did not show or call. She said that she had no idea; she wasn't thinking of me. I let her know that I was worried and concerned about her, especially since Nina has had some serious health problems that led to hospitalization in the past.

Nina was moved by my concern, and added that when she was fearful of dealing with situations that made her anxious, she did not always consider others. She was able to acknowledge the fact that she avoided uncomfortable situations rather than assert herself or confront the other person directly. This was a major issue in her marriage and in other relationships, especially with her mother. Knowing that I truly cared about her, and was not angry or disappointed as her mother and husband would have been if she stated her needs and wants, led to a deeper connection between us. Exploring this together made it possible for her to gain greater insight into herself, her relationship with others, and to experience behavioral patterns of which she was not aware.

In her relationship with her mother, Nina experienced the need to please her mother and make her proud. If she did not satisfy her mother's needs and expectations, she was rejected by her, leaving her to feel a diminished sense of self. Nina realized that she avoided our session because she was afraid I would be hurt or displeased by her desire to terminate, and that then I would disconnect from her as her mother had always done. (In effect, she rejected me before she gave me the chance to reject her.) When I didn't react the way she anticipated, she felt more validated and was more able to assert her needs.

The desire for self-assertion may engender tension when this need conflicts with girls' and women's need for security and acceptance. In her classic work, *Bonds of Love*, Jessica Benjamin (1988) concurs that tensions arise from people's need to differentiate themselves from others. Simultaneously, a fully formed self can only emerge from a supportive and close milieu, where one feels recognized and accepted. According to Benjamin, the tension between self-assertion and conformity constitutes opposite ends of a continuum, suspended in a delicate balance. Balancing both requires a paradigm shift—from an individualistic model of the self to one that allows uniqueness and difference to emerge within the context of connection. This balance is integral to what is called self-differentiation: the individual develops a self always aware of its distinctness while simultaneously needing to remain connected to others. In adolescence, this balance becomes even more precarious.

The following case example of my work with Leslie illustrates how I used myself in a relationship with a 16-year-old female adolescent who was struggling to maintain the precarious balance between her need to develop her own sense of self, and her need to conform to the expectations of others.

When I initially met Leslie, she had been living with her father and brother in a suburb of a large metropolitan area for two years. She had lived in this same town with her parents until she was three and the family decided to relocate to a small city in the Midwest. At the age of nine, Leslie's mother and father divorced and dad moved back east. For the next five years, Leslie was shuffled back and forth between her mother and father. At age 15 she permanently moved in with her father.

Leslie's mother is an alcoholic who repeatedly goes on binges, which induce paranoid episodes for which she has been hospitalized on many occasions, leaving Leslie in charge of herself and her younger brother. After the parents separated, Leslie's father discovered that the children were living with a friend's family, so he petitioned for and received custody. At Leslie's request, her father contacted the community counseling center asking for help for his daughter.

During our first session, Leslie said, "I just want someone to talk to." Although she copes well with the many stressors that impact on her life, the identity crisis most teenagers face was exacerbated by her mixed ethnicity and family instability. Dad is white and Jewish, and Mom is half white, half Native American, and Catholic. Although her father is raising Leslie as Jewish, she identifies strongly with the Native American aspect of her heritage. Most of the time Leslie feels disconnected from herself, her family, her heritage, her suburban community, her friends and family in the Midwest, and from her father, whom she frequently calls "an idiot." Until about age nine, Leslie recalls a warm and close relationship with her mother. Relying on her inner strength and early positive ties with her mother, she is quite resilient and mature, having had to grow up faster than many others her age. Her strongest connection is to her 13-year-old brother, for whom she often has had to play the role of surrogate parent.

I feel that my emotional presence is very important to Leslie. She needs someone on whom she can count to be there for her—to understand how she feels and thinks, and to acknowledge her likes and dislikes. I ask her about her music and her taste in books. We have exchanged books and CDs. Surprisingly, we like some of the same things. Leslie has a strong need to be understood and to be "recognized" by others as she struggles to integrate a coherent self-identity. In order for differentiation to evolve, Leslie needs to feel a secure attachment to another person, providing a safe mooring to launch herself into the world. Her sophisticated cognitive skills and her insight help her to see her mother and father realistically, thereby reducing self-blame, guilt, and helplessness. Our connection is based on mutual respect, honesty, and authenticity: a contrast to the hypocrisy that she feels prevails in her life.

Although part of Leslie wants to conform to an image that will earn her the approval of her peers, I continuously reinforce what is special and unique about her. Unlike the other girls in her town, she does not dress in the latest fashion, straighten her hair, nor does she paint her nails. She wears torn jeans, sneakers, and T-shirts most of the time. She likes poetry, plays the guitar, has eclectic taste in music, and likes to read books of the beat generation. In other words, she sees herself as "different," a unique individual who wants to be accepted for herself.

The need for relational resonance is great, especially for female adolescence. Girls have a strong need for connection, possibly because this is the stage in their lives where they are most likely to lose their "voice." There are many layers of the self that become submerged, hidden away from others and even from the self. Adolescent girls in particular begin to lose an authentic sense of connection because they often have not discovered their true identities (Gilligan, 1982). A good relationship with the mother or mother substitute, a pivotal figure during this stage, is still most important in helping the girl sort out the different, sometimes contrasting aspects of herself. And a secure mother–daughter relationship is one of the most significant indicators of a healthy adolescence (Kaplan et al., 1985). My position as object replacement for Leslie's mother was reparative and may have helped to offset further damage (Miller & Stiver, 1997).

Knowing the importance of the mother–daughter relationship for adolescent girls, it was difficult for me to acknowledge that Leslie did not feel she was ready to re-connect with her mom who was residing in the Midwest. She recounted that the last few times her mother telephoned she sounded drunk and had not come through on the promises she had made. Leslie was not ready to see her mother, and felt she had to protect herself from further disappointment. I shared with Leslie the fact that I respected her decision—in many ways she seemed more mature than her mother. I know the loss of such a significant relationship contributed to the feelings of loneliness and isolation she sometimes expressed, and one day she would have to deal with her relationship with her mom.

A willingness to bring observations out into the open and to elicit client feedback can provide clients with vital information about themselves and their interaction with other social systems. This is best accomplished if the worker is able to tolerate, work with, and sustain tension in the relationship. The fact that people are so complex makes it hard to predict the outcome of any helping relationship. Energy flows in many directions as long as interpersonal boundaries are permeable. The normal tension that exists in the client–worker relational system is influenced by, but not limited to the following: (1) our degree of authenticity; (2) how we regulate closeness and distance between ourselves and clients; (3) our ability to sustain connection in spite of disruption and conflict; and (4) what we do or do not disclose.

Self-disclosure

The notion of self-disclosure is related to the use of self and the concept of mutuality. Workers who adopt a more feminist relational approach agree that the more the worker shares, the more connected some clients may feel with the worker, and the more productive the relationship can be. However, according to Cooper and Lesser (2002), this "ethic of mutuality" in the therapeutic relationship does not *mandate* self-disclosure. The more traditional, psychoanalytic perspective is that worker self-disclosure is merely an attempt to gratify the client and therefore is deemed an obstacle in the therapeutic process (Raines, 1996). While this view has prevailed in some circles, as social work theory embraced systemic, ego-oriented, and interactional models, social workers themselves began to realize that there is no such thing as complete neutrality. Thus self-disclosure has received more attention and has gained wider acceptance, particularly in the feminist model of relational theory which might be more inclined to reveal parts of their authentic selves in order to connect with the client (Dewane, 2006).

The parameters of what the worker shares as opposed to what a friend, a work associate, or a family member shares are, naturally, different. Of course, selectivity is key. Be clear about what you are revealing, the reasons you are revealing it, and make it consistent with your understanding of who your client is and what they need from you. Timing is also critical. Since workers help clients mediate reality, their reactions often provide helpful feedback. Focusing on the "here and now" in the relationship can provide "*in vivo*" learning that facilitates growth and allows the client to gain a fuller recognition of how they impact others.

Sensitivity is paramount in trying to gauge how much the client can actually "hear" of the worker's negative feelings, such as disappointment or anger. More positive feelings, such as wanting to protect or care for the client, may be rejected as well, since those can be too threatening if the client has a need to maintain more formal boundaries or to reject help altogether (Miller & Stiver, 1991). Disclosure, therefore, must be based on an accurate assessment of clients and their present state of mind.

Self-disclosure is a tricky thing to negotiate. There is the fear that you may share too much, but there is also the danger of sharing too little—balance is key. Keep your client's needs in the forefront. Disclosure of the worker's experience, thoughts, and feelings is fine, but only if it serves your client—not you. Janet Surrey (1991a) suggests that not disclosing anything may have a negative effect on those clients who are prone to isolation or who have poor social skills. They may interpret this as their own failure to relate effectively or they may feel that the worker is not interested in them, resulting in a disconnection. However, the worker should not feel compelled to immediately respond to a client's request for personal information.

For example, if a client asks me if I have any children, or if I am married, or what my sexual orientation or religion is, I may answer and then explore the meaning this has for them. Sometimes I will explore the reason for their question and then choose whether or not to respond. Many times those kinds of questions are related to concerns about their own lives, or whether I can understand them and their situation, or whether there is common ground to build a relationship on. It may be very helpful, for example, for a client who is going through a divorce to know that their worker has been divorced as well. The worker can convey whatever their experience was with the intent to facilitate identification without sharing too many of the details, possibly reducing any sense of shame the client may have in the process.

If a practitioner discloses how she herself handled a particular situation, clients can feel intimidated or embarrassed, thinking that they do not have the skills to do it that way. Clients need reminding that everyone is unique and that individuals handle things differently. Disclosure must be done in a manner that helps clients learn and grow, without making them feel that they must do it *your* way. The important thing is to encourage clients to try out new behaviors compatible with who they are or who they want to be.

Then there are some clients who do not want to know anything about you. They refrain from asking any questions and seem more comfortable keeping the relationship more formal. As a general rule, social workers should avoid divulging any material that: (1) they themselves have not worked through; (2) sounds like a confession, which may make clients feel they have to protect or reassure the worker; (3) is not relevant to the helping relationship, the agency function, or that the client does not seem interested in; (4) is beyond the worker's comfort zone; and (5) is beyond the client's comfort zone.

It is important that the worker respect the client's boundaries and maintain acute sensitivity in terms of what is safe to disclose—just as in a marriage, the optimal emotional distance between two people is mutually regulated. The decision to disclose any personal information to the client is based on the assumption that the worker is able to focus on the client's needs and wants without using the client–worker situation to gratify his or her own needs. I strongly believe that the ability to exert this kind of judgment is closely related to the worker's level of maturity and self-awareness.

The case of Tracy illustrates the conscious use of self-disclosure in a manner that enhanced the client–worker relationship. Tracy is a Caucasian single mother of Justin, an 18-year-old biracial male. Her relationship with her son is a major source of pain, anger, and disappointment to Tracy. According to her they were once close, but now communication has totally broken down. She and Justin's father divorced when he was four, and Justin has not seen his dad since he was eight. At that time, the father was arrested for possession of drugs and fired from his job as a detective in the police force. Neither Tracy nor Justin ever talked about the circumstances surrounding his dad's disappearance, nor do they talk about him now. He remains the "elephant in the room." The secrecy about Justin's father has had destructive effects on everyone. As a young man trying to establish an identity in a racist world, not knowing anything about his father and his father's family is a denial of Justin's heritage and his sense of reality.

For the last two years, Justin has been using alcohol and marijuana and dealing cocaine. Most recently he was arrested for possession of marijuana. It appears that Justin harbors a deep need for an attachment with his biological father, demonstrated by the fact that his behavior replicates that of his father. According to Miller and Stiver (1995), individuals like Justin often become fearful of becoming close to others because of past neglect, humiliation, and loss. In response, they begin to isolate parts of themselves, and develop a repertoire of strategies that keep others at a distance—safe enough from being hurt again.

According to Tracy, Justin is opposed to any request she makes of him, even one as small as having dinner together on Sunday evenings. She feels he is "just a boarder" in the house. The reality of raising a difficult adolescent is overwhelming to her. The sense of helplessness she feels is contrary to her usual self-image of a competent woman in control of her life. What Tracy perceives as a loss of power or failure in her maternal role she has turned against herself. She has not gone out socially in years, has not invested in her community, nor has she done much of anything to feel good about herself.

Although she presents as a stoic, independent woman, Tracy actually feels hurt, unloved, lonely, and frustrated. She has few social connections or supports. Tracy has invested her whole life in Justin, and feels a deep sense of shame in believing she has failed as a parent. This has caused her to further isolate herself from friends and family.

Taking on the responsibility to meet the needs of others begins at birth, often leading women to become more "other-focused." The implications of this are two-fold: (1) women have been trained to look to others for affirmation and value, placing them in a vulnerable position; and (2) women have been given the message by society that self-denial is characteristic of good mothering. Yet if one ignores one's own needs, the anger connected to depriving the self may accumulate and initiate a cycle of inadequate mothering and low self-esteem for both mother and child. Both Tracy and Justin were caught in this cycle.

I thought about my own adolescence—how I had rebelled against my parents in an effort to establish a clearer sense of self. I shared this with Tracy, which led us to talk about the ways in which she rebelled against her parents during adolescence. Through this discussion, I was hoping that she could gain a greater degree of empathy for her son. Although Tracy desperately wanted a closer relationship with Justin, she was not able to see how her anger pushed him away. Without realizing it, she was creating a situation in which she disconnected from Justin, he then disconnected from her, and both experienced a vicious cycle of rejection.

Tracy and I talked about her disappointment and pain. I commented that if she and Justin were to have any relationship at all, approaching him in an angry manner would only further humiliate and alienate him. I suggested that it may be best to express her own feelings of hurt and disappointment to let him know how much she wanted to be a part of his life, rather than give in to the impulse to cut herself off or react out of anger. I shared my experience with my own adolescent children and said that when I was vulnerable and open, they responded in kind. Also, no matter how angry or hurt I was, I always tried to remember that I was the grown-up and had to make the first move when communication broke down.

I did let Tracy know that it was hard for me at times, and maybe for her too, to be the "adult" with our teenage children. I said, "When we are hurt or feel rejected, our impulse is to lash out and hurt back, but that just creates more obstacles." Communicating with Tracy in this more personal way modeled how she could be more open with Justin to engage in a freer give and take. I conveyed my belief that if she revealed more about herself—her thoughts, her disappointments, her experiences—to her son, she would come across as more approachable and accessible. In turn, Justin might respond more openly to her.

As our relationship grew over time, Tracy gradually made significant changes, which in turn had an impact on Justin. For example, with my support Tracy began to connect with others, which helped reduce her isolation. I encouraged her to talk with her sister-in-law who was in recovery. She understood Tracy's situation and could offer her the support she needed. Tracy's two brothers also got involved, so Justin now had two adult male figures with whom he could relate in the absence of his father. Tracy also joined a parent self-help support group, and to her surprise, connected with many of the other group members. The relationships with her family and members of the group helped her to feel more secure and to set more consistent limits for Justin.

As Tracy became closer with members of her parents' group, she was afforded the opportunity to share similar experiences in an atmosphere of mutuality. She was able to give to others and get back in return. This was rewarding for Tracy, and she began to seek out more connections and felt part of a larger community. She became a volunteer at the city performing arts center and was thinking of working in a local political campaign. Now that she was meeting people, was more connected to her own community, and had more of her own life, she could relax her hold on Justin. Reciprocally, Justin began to feel that he could more comfortably move closer to his mom as they developed a new and different relationship together.

Relational authenticity

What is meant by relational authenticity? Working in a relational way and using the authentic self implies that the worker participates in a relationship in which he or she feels comfortable enough in the presence of the other to be "real." Thus, the practitioner's verbalizations and actions will hopefully be congruent and conducive to engaging the client in a relationship that facilitates trust and growth (Miller et al. 1999).

According to Jean Baker Miller and Irene Stiver (1997), the worker's disclosure of true feelings, selective sharing of experiences, lack of defensiveness, and presentation of a less-than-perfect authority promotes a sense of relational authenticity that can be the impetus for a real exchange. Instead of stressing the importance of neutrality, the client–worker relationship is more productive when the worker is authentically present and participating in the relationship with the client as an equal or "near equal" partner.

The following example illustrates the importance of the worker's ability to remain open to differences of all kinds—cultural, class, gender, sexual orientation, and value systems. Nancy is a 35-year-old, second-generation Latina woman. She is highly intelligent and successful in her career as a pharmacist. Her competence in the work place enabled her to recently get a raise and a promotion. Her fiancé Tony, a 45-year-old, second-generation Italian man, is much more traditional and expects his wife-to-be to assume the same roles and responsibilities in their home as his mother had. Although Nancy is willing to go along with this to a point, she expressed doubts about their long-term compatibility. She was willing to do a good deal of the domestic tasks but did not want this to undermine her career.

Nancy knew that being a traditional housewife like Tony's mom would not quite fit her, but she really wanted to marry. She was emotionally dependent on Tony, loved him, and believed she could be happy with him. She asked me what I thought. I stated that different household arrangements work best for different couples; the reality of her experience is that she might have to compromise her ideas of gender equality if she wanted to have a long-term relationship with Tony.

I related to Nancy that like many women, I too have struggled with dependency needs. Being authentic involves being true to your values and ideals without judging another. I thought that it was important to help Nancy examine her own feelings about gender roles and whether she would be comfortable adjusting her ideals and assuming the role of housewife to achieve her desire for security and marriage. I let Nancy know that I thought it was very important that she make a decision that best fit her needs and wishes and those of her fiancé rather than what I believed or anyone else for that matter. I also wondered if she thought there might be room for negotiation and compromise. I believed that my role was to help her clarify the extent to which she was willing to accommodate to difference or negotiate conflict without losing self-esteem or a sense of control over her life.

This notion of authenticity has many implications for the way the clinician uses him or herself in the relationship. When we are fully present with the client, we can move with greater ease. When we are in touch with our own feelings, thoughts, and intuitions—our true selves—we are moving toward becoming more integrated, more authentic workers; something which continues as we mature into our professional roles through training, supervision, and commitment to our own growth. The feminist relational notion of authenticity is congruent with many of the basic notions presented in the social work literature. Hepworth et al. (2006) define it as "the sharing of the self by relating in a natural, sincere, spontaneous, open, and genuine manner" (p. 107). Being authentic or genuine involves relating personally to the other so that expressions are spontaneous rather than contrived. Although the worker can be naturally spontaneous, both perception and judgment are always modified by professional training. It is important to remember that spontaneity is not the same as being impulsive, the later being more of an unpredictable response without regard for consequences. Spontaneity, rather, is an unguarded, unconstrained, unforced, and unaffected response. Direct and spontaneous articulation of the worker's feelings is acceptable as long as it is not based on the worker's own needs, but rather guided by therapeutic intention.

As social workers, we are trained to use ourselves in an egalitarian way, which means that we are keenly aware of redistributing as much of the power in the relationship as possible, given the parameters of our role. Regardless of setting, the feminist relational approach dictates that one is, above all, honest and open about purpose, goals, and possible outcomes of the helping process, thereby maximizing the principle of self-determination. Sometimes the worker will make an error, a poorly timed inter-vention perhaps, resulting in the client disconnecting. Whatever the precipitating factor, mistakes are inevitable.

It is the willingness and responsibility of the worker to at least explore what hap-pened and attempt to repair any damage that are most important. The goal is to move from disconnection to connection without the client disengaging from or disrupting the relationship. In essence, the social worker must be willing to learn from the client and be able to admit when he or she has made a mistake.

The role of transference–countertransference in the relational model

In the 1950s and 1960s, Helen Harris Perlman (1957) and Florence Hollis (1964) cautioned social workers to maintain firm boundaries in the service of controlling transference and countertransference reactions, thinking that the expression of these could distort the relationship. Now that we have moved toward using ourselves in a more open way, the way in which we understand transference phenomena needs to be reframed. Originally associated with Freudian theory, the term transference refers to the transfer of earlier unresolved feelings about some significant persons in the past onto the client-therapist relationship. In other words, it is a repetition in the present of a relationship that was important in a person's childhood (Franz, 1963).

When viewed in a relational context, transference phenomena are part of a norma-tive, therapeutic process. It is not unusual that a social worker in a helping role would remind the client of someone who has been significant in his or her life. It becomes the worker's responsibility to guide the client in exploring, understanding, and "giving voice" to these feelings and thoughts. Many times the "mysterious" notion of trans-ference is accessible to consciousness and can be used for increased insight about how we relate to other people.

Miller and Stiver (1997) seek to differentiate the emotional responses that are anchored in the past, and which are more reflective of the present relationship between worker and client. Sometimes this is difficult to determine since, realistically, things are not purely one or the other, but a mixture of both. The more self-aware one strives to be, the better chance one has at distinguishing the two. Sometimes it is helpful to discuss memories of one's past relationships in the context of safety, particularly if these memories evoke strong feelings such as anger, fear, or love. We all elicit feelings in each other, and it is important not to negate this, but rather to process them so clients can learn how to deal with their feelings in constructive ways (Wishnie, 2005). By working in the transference, the client can be helped to gain a greater understanding of past relationships in which distortions and misunderstand-ings have led to disconnection.

In classical Freudian psychoanalytic theory, countertransference represents feelings and wishes for an object of the past that are projected onto the client. In contem-porary psychodynamic theory and practice, countertransference encompasses all the thoughts, feelings, fantasies, reactions, dreams, and other responses of the helper toward the one being helped (Cooper & Lesser, 2005).

In the relational view, countertransference includes anything that helps or hurts a therapist's ability to maintain a real connection with a client—to be truly present and truly aware. Rather than see it as an impediment, countertransference can be an opportunity for the social worker to learn more about the client by examining all the thoughts and feelings stirred up in the interaction (Miller & Stiver, 1991, 1997). Much of the time the practitioner is picking up on feelings the client is experiencing and cannot acknowledge. Once aware of these dynamics, he or she can be more empathic and responsive to the client's distress.

The following case illustrates the worker's ability to balance acceptance of the client and an understanding of the transference while setting limits on unacceptable behavior. I had been seeing Michael, a white, 34-year-old man, for about six months for issues related to job performance and relationship problems. Upon returning from the bathroom during one session, Michael's zipper was open and his penis was exposed. I felt uncomfortable but decided it was important to comment on this and said, "I don't know if you are aware, but you did not close your zipper when you re-entered the office." Michael said he was sorry and got up to do so. I asked how he felt when I confronted him because he looked ruffled. He disclosed that he purposely had been exposing himself to women for years. He liked to "take them by surprise" and got a thrill out of embarrassing them. The irony is that Michael suffered from shame his whole life due to an over-controlling critical mother. His father in turn was verbally demeaning and abusive to his mother. He did not understand why she could not stand up to him. His anger at women came out in the only way he felt he could control them—to scare and shame them as *he* had been. I was another female authority figure who he feared could shame him as his mother had.

I did not feel angry or uncomfortable once I brought his behavior patterns to his attention. In fact, I felt relieved. I believe Michael was also relieved that his secret was revealed. I shared with Michael how much I appreciated his honesty, and was glad he was willing to work on his issues with me. But he needed clear boundaries and limit setting, and I let him know that I would not tolerate any more acting out.

Boundaries

According to Judith Jordan, boundaries are often depicted in traditional literature as a means of protection rather than as potential avenues of exchange. The boundaried self is restricted in openness and emotional responsiveness (Jordan, 1984). A frequent criticism of feminist-oriented relational theories involves the notion of boundaries. Traditional approaches hold that a clear separation between worker and client maintains professionalism and averts over-involvement. I prefer to see boundaries established by continuous and natural interaction. On one hand, most clients usually have some need to make contact with each other, on the other hand, they also have a need to protect themselves and maintain distance. As trust is built, and degrees of closeness are regulated, natural boundaries are established from working together and sharing intimate moments.

What distinguishes the relational approach from other models is the belief that boundaries can represent a place of meeting rather than a line of demarcation (Jordan & Dooley, 2000). The relational perspective stresses that because individuals thrive when they engage in growth-fostering relationships, client–worker boundaries need to be flexible to allow for the flow of reciprocal energy that empowers and encourages client participation (Jordan, 1991d).

Contrary to a more traditional psychodynamic approach in which there is overt concern about maintaining emotional distance, the relational social worker allows for a wide range of feelings and thoughts in the moment, facilitating a sense of connection

(Jordan, 1984). However, feeling deeply with the other is not the same thing as "merger," nor does it suggest a "blurring of the self with the other," as some male theorists have suggested. Although boundaries may be regulated by both client and worker depending on the setting, the reality is that workers can set limits based on their assessment of the client and his or her needs. Clearly, boundaries are helpful in providing safety. But flexibility and permeability allow the worker to emphasize and respect the vulnerability of the other.

At times, there might even be a sense of "fusion" between client and worker, although this does not necessarily mean a loss of boundaries. According to Berzoff (1989), females found to be at the highest levels of ego development described the phenomenon of fusion in their closest friendships. This indicates a deep ability for closeness, but at the same time, a clear sense of self in relation to the other. Perhaps a state of interdependence would be ideal, one in which healthy dependency needs are accepted, fluid, shared, and mutually met, while each person maintains a strong sense of self in a relational context of trust and intimacy.

Dependency

Some clients require a greater degree of dependency than others, for example, the frail elderly, those in crisis, and children. Inherent in all of us is a striving toward autonomy, and the push toward growth usually supersedes the wish to remain helpless. Negotiating the tendency between dependence and independence is necessary and is to be respected, not faulted. The worker's emotional and physical availability (similar to those of a parent) can provide a corrective emotional experience. As the individual matures, dependency needs remain part of every relationship in some form. Sometimes the worker has to help the client learn to be dependent on them while working incrementally toward increasing autonomy, especially when the client needs emotional support and replenishment in preparation for more independent functioning in the future.

Irene Stiver (1991c) defines dependency as "a process counting on other people to provide help in coping, physically and emotionally, with the experiences and tasks encountered in the world when one has not sufficient skill, confidence, energy, and/or time" (p. 160). Her definition stresses dependency not as a static condition, but rather one that changes along with opportunities and circumstances, making an ongoing assessment all the more important.

Dependency has to do with relying on something or someone else for support, and is not a condition that is held in high esteem in our individualistic culture. Yet for some clients whose basic needs were not met early on, it may be absolutely essential to encourage dependency. In fact, it is difficult to become independent without first having been dependent to a certain degree. Dependency is not a value-free concept. In our individualistic society that extols self-reliance, the word carries pejorative connotations of weakness, vulnerability, helplessness. Whereas the male-constructed ethic of self-reliance, independence, and individualism has permeated our cultural ideas, men and women are encouraged to discard or conceal rather than acknowledge feelings of dependency, or the need for attachment, caring, and support.

In the process of forming relationships, dependency is often labeled as an expression of regressive needs (Miller, 1976). However, in the feminist relational approach, dependency is not seen as inherently regressive, nor does being dependent necessarily equal losing the ability to cope. Women's affiliative needs do not preclude their ability to maintain a consolidated identity, nor do men's independent maneuvers preclude their need for connection. To compensate for cultural bias, the worker must respect the dependency needs of all clients and accept and regard these non-judgmentally.

Feminist thinkers such as Carol Gilligan (1982) have noted a cultural bias against permitting and encouraging dependence. Gilligan discusses the differences in how dependency issues are experienced by women and men. Men have more social pressure to disown their dependency needs. As a consequence, they often keep their distance from others to avoid being "reeled in." The idea that men have more difficulties in acknowledging their need for others than women has caught the attention of several other theorists. Dorothy Dinnerstein (1997) takes the position that a man's effort to achieve a sexual identity different from his mother propels him to repudiate levels of autonomous functioning.

Social work best practices for building the client–worker relationship

A social worker you can strengthen the client–worker relationship through practicing a number of proven techniques:

- The client–worker relationship serves as a model for other relationships. The social worker has the opportunity to use the relationship as a restorative experience for the client.
- The social worker must be genuine and congruent at all times, expressing commitment and a sense of caring on a consistent basis.
- Mutuality is critical to the client–worker relationship. The social work clinician must facilitate a reciprocal exchange of feelings and thoughts between worker and client.
- The social work clinician focuses on significant disconnections as well as connections in the client's life space; especially, those relationships which impede or enhance the client's ability to feel empowered.
- The desire and yearning for relational ties with others is strong throughout the life cycle and impacts the way clients deal with stress, trauma, and normative phases of human growth and development. The social worker seeks to mobilize positive relational networks, relational ties, and exchanges in the environment to enhance clients' coping capacities.

In summary, the mutual exchange that occurs between the client system and worker is made possible by the capacity of each participant for mutuality, mutual respect, emotional availability, relational responsiveness and awareness, openness to being moved by the other, and mutual empathy.

The intersectionality of relational theory with trauma theory

Relational theory and trauma theory can be complementary frameworks when working with the victim of a traumatic incident. Traumatic events often produce relational ruptures. Developing a safe, trusting relationship in a non-threatening environment with the clinician is crucial in helping the client cope with life's stresses. It enables the client to restructure relational patterns in relationships outside of the therapeutic dyad. According to Stone Center psychiatrist Amy Banks, a sense of safety in the relationship can be re-established by the clinician (2006).

The case of Natalie illustrates the clinician's best practices for building a strong client–worker relationship using relational concepts as discussed in this chapter—relational authenticity, the role of transference and countertransference, mutuality, and self-disclosure. The following case is illustrative of type 1 trauma: a single discrete event of catastrophic proportions, such as natural disasters, witnessing and/or experiencing a violent or potentially life threatening and dangerous act, death, accident, and the loss of family, friends, cultural tradition, community and property due to refugee status (Herman, 1997).

Natalie is a 35-year-old white female who was pregnant with her first child when she came to the counseling center because she needed help managing her anxiety. She was assigned to a female therapist who was in her early thirties, white, and from a similar socioeconomic background. Natalie was experiencing anxiety attacks on a fairly regular basis. She had worked with other therapists in the past to deal with this problem; however, her decision to re-engage in therapy was fueled primarily by the impending arrival of her first child and her desire to abate her symptoms of anxiety without psychotropic medication. Natalie also feared the responsibility that came with being a mother, as well as the increased stress which may prevent her from bonding with her child.

At the age of eight, Natalie experienced a traumatic incident. Her history revealed that her mother, father, brother, and herself were robbed at gunpoint in her family home by two intruders while they forced her father to open the home safe and hand over money and jewelry. They then tied them up in the living room where they remained until they were discovered by a neighbor the following day. They were questioned by the police but the robbers were never apprehended.

Natalie lived in a small Midwestern city where her family owned a department store in the community, a well-known fact that made them vulnerable to attack.

Four years after the incident, her father received a phone call saying that if he did not hand over a large sum of money he and the rest of his family would be harmed. He immediately called the police and arranged a sting operation at the agreed-upon meeting place. But the extortionists never showed up and the case remained unsolved. The family lived with a looming sense of fear for years to come. After these two incidents, and basically throughout her childhood and adolescence, Natalie's parents were constantly fearful for her safety and transmitted this anxiety to Natalie and her brother. She described her parents as hyper-vigilant; they installed an elaborate alarm system, rarely left Natalie and her brother alone, and developed contingency plans for escape should they feel in danger again.

Natalie has been married for three years and lives with her husband in an apartment in a mid-size city about 120 miles from her mother, father, and brother. She has kept her anxiety attacks a secret from her parents and brother, in part because of the shame she feels, and in part because she does not want to cause them worry. She also has difficulties being vulnerable with her husband; the anxiety attacks often come when her husband is away on business and Natalie is alone at night. At first she saw no relationship between her anxiety attacks and the traumatic events of her childhood. In fact, she laughed when referring to the incidents saying it was "no big deal," and made clear that she did not want to discuss them in treatment.

Natalie's attempts to numb herself from the early trauma enabled her to function fairly successfully; she is professionally accomplished, is married to a kind and considerate man, and has a few friends. However, her relationships are compromised when it comes to the degree of intimacy she is able to tolerate, fearing her "secret" would surface if she exposed her "true self." Emotionally, she remained a frightened little girl who needed protection. Natalie's anxiety contributes to a constant state of hyper-vigilance, a high level of tension and stress, manifesting in physical symptoms such as headaches, accelerated heart rate, palpitations, and sweating.

Natalie describes herself as a "type A" personality; she runs 5–6 miles a day, and has a demanding job which frequently requires multi-tasking in order to successfully complete concurrent projects. She feels pressure to appear "perfect" and tries to remain "cheerful" (or be the "good girl") most times. Although she reports that her family remains a major source of emotional support, she is reluctant to share negative feelings and thoughts with them, thus keeping her true self hidden.

Natalie's history of trauma has affected her ability to fully connect with others. She initially presented herself as self-reliant and conflicted about asking for help. Many individuals who have experienced some trauma may enter treatment unaware of their needs and how to negotiate them in the therapeutic dyad as well as outside of it (Banks, 2006).

A good deal of the clinician's work with Natalie focused on her desire to please others, and how this behavior may be connected to her anxiety and trauma history. Goals for treatment included: (1) better management of Natalie's current anxiety; (2) recognizing the impact of her trauma history on her behavior; and (3) developing a reparative therapeutic relationship. The worker borrowed from both a relational–cultural approach and a phase oriented trauma model to help decrease anxiety attacks, and to help Natalie integrate her early life experience with her current situation. The work of the clinician focused on engaging Natalie in a relationship where she could express her needs and feelings, and to help her feel safe in an atmosphere of mutuality, care, and trust.

Discussion—phase-oriented trauma model and relational themes

The case of Natalie is a good illustration of the intersection of relational theory and phase specific trauma theory developed by Judith Herman (1997). In phase-oriented work, the clinician first works with phase 1 objectives: safety and stabilization. By engaging Natalie in a supportive relationship where she felt accepted by the therapist who could hold and regulate her own feelings, Natalie eventually became less fearful and more willing to address the traumatic life event.

Initially, Natalie was uncomfortable talking with the worker; giving up control and admitting her vulnerabilities was difficult. She was unable to describe her anxiety attacks: when she experienced them, their frequency, duration, and intensity, her thoughts and feelings during the attacks, and what triggered them. She had limited awareness of her physical or emotional states, and was unable to effectively regulate her emotions when feeling distressed. She maintained a hyper-vigilant protective stance, which took a toll on her body as well as on her relationships with her husband, friends, and family.

During one session early on Natalie appeared particularly anxious: she was tense, had trouble concentrating, and was hyperventilating. Initially, she had no awareness of this presentation. However, during the discussion she revealed that her husband was traveling for work that evening and she would be home alone for two nights. She identified feeling frightened, worried, and abandoned, but was not able to make the connection between her anxiety and her physical sensations.

The therapist displayed attunement by observing the client's distress and reflecting this back in a concerned, caring manner—interventions which helped to create a proper *holding environment* (Winnicott, 1965); a milieu in which Natalie could feel safe enough to reveal her true thoughts and feelings and a more authentic self. The worker maintained appropriate boundaries and adopted an open, relaxed, and caring attitude, minimizing the power differential, helping Natalie take a greater sense of agency rather than duplicating the passive–helpless stance she sometimes assumed.

Over the course of treatment the worker and client were able to develop a sense of mutuality. Coincidentally, as a youngster, the clinician herself had been a victim of an armed robbery, an experience that allowed her to tap into her own memories and authentically demonstrate a sense of empathy. The worker had decided not to disclose her experience, believing it would not move the work forward, but she was able to use it and respond in a genuinely helpful manner, saying, "When I hear about your experiences, I can understand how this must have had a lasting impact on you as a young child. It sounds like from what you are telling me, you stood there frozen in terror, knowing that you could not do anything to help yourself or your family."

Transference is a relational phenomenon which emerges in all relationships. In the relational view, the therapist is not merely a blank screen but a genuine, supportive, and empathic figure who may provide a relational context in which both patient and therapist become acutely aware of older relational images as they are expressed in the transference. Here, the worker helped the patient to use the therapeutic relationship in order to experience an intimate relationship in a way that enabled the client to be more "herself," without having to take care of the other. The worker is well advised to use her awareness of her own feelings to identify with and better understand the client, and to communicate thoughts and feelings.

The worker's facial expression, tone, and posture conveyed her deep sense of compassion. Natalie said: "I try not to think about it or talk about it. It is easier to pretend it's no big deal. But I can see from your response that other people may view if differently." The worker said: "I can see how hard it is for you. You don't have to say any more now if you don't want to, but over time, it would be helpful to share your thoughts and feelings about this with me so I can fully understand what this experience was like for you and so you can one day feel more comfortable acknowledging it too."

The worker conveyed to Natalie that she was moved by her experience. Natalie could feel the impact she was having on the worker, and the clinician could see the impact she was having on the client. Out of an atmosphere of mutual respect and concern, Natalie started to develop a sense of trust in the worker and in the therapeutic process. Over time, the clinician's ability to empathetically "sit with" the client and "hold" her anxiety enabled Natalie to become less fearful; she was gradually able to remember and talk about the traumatic event in detail.

The focus of the second phase—remembrance and mourning—was to establish a narrative of the trauma. The role of the worker here, similar to the first phase, is to provide a safe environment, one in which Natalie could talk in more detail about the traumatic experience itself, physically experience it differently, and learn how to exert more control over her anxiety. To facilitate this, the clinician used "grounding" techniques. Each week she began their session by asking Natalie to observe the treatment room—its smells, images on the walls, the windows, and any physical or emotional sensations she felt. Initially this was difficult for Natalie since she was unaccustomed to taking much notice of her environment; she did not have the words or language to describe many of her feelings. But with practice, she had more tools at her disposal and awareness.

For example, she eventually allowed herself to notice the sturdiness of the chair, the brightness of the light shining through the window, the warm colors of the walls and the furniture, and the calming scent that permeated the room. She identified a wall hanging of a flower in the office as a grounding image. If she felt destabilized when narrating her trauma, she would return to these images and sensations to bring her back to the present. This became a safe image for her throughout treatment. The worker would ask her to feel her feet on the ground, her back against the chair, and her own physical responses. Her ability to notice these sensations and enhance her physical awareness was integral to our work and to helping her improve her ability to establish a sense of safety in the outside world.

In the third phase, reconnection and reintegration, the client–worker relationship assumes central focus. The goal is to eliminate behavior that is dysfunctional and provide the client with psycho-education and concrete skills with which to build stability in everyday life by managing symptoms and enhancing social support. The clinician was able to facilitate a mutual and authentic exchange of feelings, identify with Natalie's traumatic experience, and stay within her own boundaries while simultaneously being open to the emotional experiences of the client. With the support of a mutual, respectful relationship with the worker, Natalie stated that she did not feel so alone anymore. Feeling relatively safe, she was able to lift the veil of denial that had isolated her from her own self as well as others. Her increased sense of connectedness enabled her to risk sharing her vulnerabilities making it easier to move toward more intimate connections with family, her husband, and friends.

The client–worker relationship became a model for healthy relationships with others. Basic education about what constitutes a growth-fostering relationship both in and out of therapy is important as Natalie did not really know what to expect from relationships. The worker and Natalie discussed the "five good things" that would ideally follow from authentic engagement in mutual relationships: (1) an increased sense of energy within the relationship; (2) more satisfying connection with the other; (3) a greater sense of clarity about the self and the other; (4) each person within the relationship has a greater sense of worth; and (5) an enhanced sense of self-esteem (Miller & Stiver, 1997). Natalie's relationship with the worker enabled her to develop an increased desire to engage with others in relationships that are more authentic and growth-fostering than before she began therapy; she is not as afraid to encounter difference and deal with conflict.

Implications for best practices that can be drawn from the case of Natalie in stage focused trauma-relational work are:

- the use of self as part of a grounding technique to establish a safe environment in the stage of safety and stabilization;
- the provision of empathic responses to engender mutuality in the remembrance stage of trauma focused work; and

- the development of the therapeutic relationship as a model of a safe relationship in the stage of reconnection and mourning.

In summary, the mutual exchange that occurs between the client system and worker is made possible by the capacity of each participant for mutuality, mutual respect, emotional availability, relational responsiveness and awareness, openness to being moved by the other, and mutual empathy. In the next chapter we will explore the notion of mutual empathy as a particularly significant relational aspect of the social work relationship.

4 Relational theory and empathy
A relational–cultural perspective

For thousands of years, people have been aware of what is now commonly referred to as *empathy*. In ancient Greece, philosophers expressed their understanding with the word *empatheia*, which implies an active appreciation of another person's feeling experience (Astin, 1967). The English word derives from the German *Einfuhlung*, which literally means "feeling oneself into." Empathy was introduced into our clinical vocabulary by German psychologist Edward Tichener at the turn of the twentieth century and was generally accepted as the equivalent of *Einfuhlung* (Berger, 1987). Almost every modern conceptualization of the word shares the notion that empathy involves the capacity to participate in the inner experience of another or to comprehend the feelings or ideas of another.

Throughout the twentieth century social workers have been influenced by Freudian and ego-oriented theorists in their understanding and application of empathy. Freud conceived of empathy as a cognitive technique that enhanced the therapist's ability to enter into the internal world of the client, thereby facilitating accurate interpretation of unconscious material (Bohart & Greenberg, 1997). By exploring the patient's thoughts and feelings without judging them, the use of empathy could help the therapist gain insight into the patient's motivation. Despite Freud's use of empathy as an intrapsychic process, he generally regarded it as a background variable with limited curative powers.

In more classical psychoanalytic thinking, the therapist is expected to suppress any and all feelings evoked by the patient in order to avoid countertransference (Basch, 1988). It was thought that communicating emotionality might distort the neutrality of the relationship and impede the development of the transference. So it was considered best that the clinician remain a passive listener and convey a neutral, objective stance (Bohart & Greenberg, 1997).

Some psychoanalytically minded theorists consider empathy, along with subjectivity, suspended rationality, and emotionality, to be distinctly feminine traits. A parallel has been made between a worker's empathy for a client and a mother's empathy for her child, reaffirming a tie to the female role, one often devalued in our society (Berger, 1987). When social work incorporated modern psychodynamic theories into its knowledge base from the 1950s through the 1970s—ego psychology, client-centered theory, self-psychology, and object relations theory—the emphasis shifted from drive theory to the role of the relational milieu in producing and reproducing healthy growth and development. It was during this time that empathy came to play a more central role in social work practice.

Relational contexts: psychological metaphors for empathy

Object relations theorist D.W. Winnicott (1965) considered empathy and emotional attunement to be *the* most crucial elements in mothering, which suggests a parallel between the "good enough" mother and the "good enough" social worker. According to Winnicott, the mother's anticipation of her baby's needs and the proper timing in meeting those needs are the basis for the development of a healthy, creative self. Similarly, through the use of empathy, the worker provides a facilitating environment for growth, development, and the enhancement of adaptive skills. If, in the safety of the therapeutic environment, the client experiences the worker as empathic and accepting, it is more likely that an authentic self will unfold, setting the stage for a more trusting relationship with the worker (Greenberg & Mitchell, 1983).

Fox (2001) calls this protective therapeutic milieu the "safe house," a place where the social worker supplies some of the nurturance missing from the client's earlier experience. Through the use of empathy, the social worker's task is to enable clients to feel understood and accepted enough to risk revealing hidden parts of themselves. Simultaneously, the worker relaxes his/her own boundaries, so that the reaction clients evoke in the clinician become more readily accessible. It is this kind of relational "holding" that maximizes the therapeutic value of empathy and has the potential for far-reaching interpersonal change.

Carl Rogers (1951), the father of client-centered therapy, identified empathy as "the ability to perceive the internal frame of reference of another with accuracy without ever losing the 'as if' condition" (p. 210). According to Rogers, empathy is not only used as a means to an end, but also as an end in itself, and involves a focus on understanding the subtleties of the client's experience in the moment. It is the clinician's attempts to reflect understanding of the client's world that remain at the core of the healing process.

Kohut (1977) views the capacity to empathize as a cornerstone of the development of an integrated sense of self. His school of self-psychology stresses the primacy of the worker's ability to understand, and then reflect on, the client's subjective experience. Kohut defines empathy as "the capacity to experience the patient's inner life while remaining objective" (p. 16). Mirroring the client's reality—feelings, thoughts, experiences, and perceptions—helps build a cohesive sense of self (Greenberg & Mitchell, 1983). Thus, empathic responses on the part of the clinician can create a milieu that potentially compensates for repeated empathic failures in childhood; those moments when the caretaker did not tune in and respond in an accurate and timely manner to the child's wants and needs (Eisenberg & Strayer, 1987).

Contemporary definitions and characteristics

Many social work theorists consider empathy as central to human experience and a critical element in professional practice (Hepworth et al., 2006; Germain & Gitterman, 1986; Raines, 1990). Keefe (1976) defines it as a "set of behaviors that constitute a skill central to effective social work intervention at every level" (p. 10). It has also been referred to as "the ability of the practitioner to understand, as accurately as possible, what it is that a client is experiencing from the client's frame of reference" (Boyle et al., 2006, p. 113). Although social work scholars conceptualize empathy somewhat differently, all highlight the same essential elements:

- active listening;
- genuineness and positive regard;
- a sense of understanding; and
- accurate attunement to emotional and cognitive processes.

Most social workers recognize that without empathy, there would be fewer engaged clients and fewer successful outcomes. Studies consistently identify empathy as one of the critical variables affecting the helping process and closely correlated with effective outcomes in social work practice. For example, Truax and Mitchell (1971) found a direct correlation between the therapist's empathy, warmth, and genuineness, and client change. Shulman (2006) corroborates these findings, citing empathy as a powerful ingredient in building a constructive working relationship.

Conveying empathy

For most social workers, empathy involves not only the ability to enter into the experience of another, but also the ability to communicate that understanding and create an atmosphere of validation and support. Once demonstrated, the client may be more likely to trust that the clinician is there to help and, as a result, may work harder and more collaboratively.

Although Woods and Hollis (1999) view empathy as an essential element in demonstrating a sense of caring for the client and enhancing his or her feeling of being understood and respected, they recommend at the same time that clinicians contain their own feelings. Their position is that if social workers do not harness their own personal responses, those responses could potentially interfere with the client's own process and ultimately circumvent transference reactions.

In standard social work practice, empathy is generally used descriptively and in conjunction with other basic skills, such as reflection and clarification—with the caveat that the social worker should not focus too intensely on the client's affective state nor take on the emotions experienced by the client as the clinician's own. According to Hepworth and his colleagues (2006), the first dimension of clinical practice, *recognition*, involves mainly insight and cognition, keeping in mind that there is growing empirical data that there is a relationship between emotions, cognition, and behavior. The second, *demonstration*, is a comprehension of the client's inner experience through accurate reflection of thoughts and feelings.

While empathic communication involves "stepping into the shoes" of the other, Hepworth et al. argue that the clinician must simultaneously remain outside of the client's inner emotional world "to avoid being overwhelmed by his or her fears, angers, joys, and hurts" (2006, p. 87). Accordingly, these authors do not believe the worker should focus too intensely on the client's affective state, or take on the emotions experienced by the client as if those were the worker's own, since it might result in the worker losing his/her own perspective, thus reducing the ability to be helpful.

Much of the traditional literature suggests that social workers should never abandon neutrality (Keefe, 1976; Raines, 1990). This idea implies that retaining separateness is a critically important dimension in the helping process. According to Keefe: "Empathy is the worker's understanding of the feelings the other has about the situation, knowing inside oneself how uncomfortable and desperate these feeling may be for the client, but never claiming these feelings for oneself as the helping person" (1976, pp. 30–31).

Compton et al. (2005, p. 151) best capture what social workers see as its inherent tensions and contradictions: "Empathy requires what may seem to many beginning workers to be antithetical qualities—the capacity to feel emotion deeply and yet to remain separate enough from it to be able to use [that] knowledge."

Social workers who embrace a more traditional psychoanalytic view often err on the side of maintaining too much distance, thereby making it difficult to fully engage in a satisfying relationship: one in which the client is able to trust that the worker is genuinely "there." Modern-day workers are cautioned to maintain clear and separate boundaries so as to avoid the possibility of over-identifying with the client. It is here that the relational–cultural model and mainstream social work approach to empathy part ways.

One of the basic differences between traditional social work practice and the feminist approach is the degree to which the practitioner remains "outside" the client's experience. Keen self-awareness and the ability to maintain clear yet flexible boundaries are the most important ingredients in being able to resonate deeply with the feelings and experiences of the client while remaining closely connected to one's own feelings and experiences.

While traditional concepts of empathy call for the worker to understand the client and to express his or her understanding, feminist relational theorists conceptualize this phenomenon more broadly, as a reciprocal, dynamic process, embedded in the client–worker relational/cultural context, growing and changing over time. The worker who expresses empathy in the form of interest in and concern for the other serves as a role model in helping clients learn ways to enhance all of their relationships—with family, with friends, and with members of their communities. Similar to the ideas of Carl Rogers (1951), feminist relational theorists believe that empathy provides a secure and safe context that validates and reaffirms the client's sense of self. Thus, empathy in the therapeutic process increases the client's ability to feel free to be his/her "true self" in the presence of another (Stiver & Miller, 1988).

The intersubjective approach

Jessica Benjamin (1988) offers a relational model that considers empathy from an intersubjective point of view; that is, the client and worker regard each other's subjective states from their separate vantage points. The notion of *intersubjectivity* implies a high level of emotional attunement and sharing, and can serve as an instrument of therapeutic change. Both client and clinician recognize that they have an impact on the other, are intent on learning more about themselves and the other, and can grow from the experience of working together. According to Benjamin, through the empathic, confirming response of the therapist, the client comes to feel recognized, affirmed, and valued.

This recognition implies that the worker and the client have entered into each other's emotional world, thereby reducing the distance between them. The worker is not seen as merely an object of the client's needs, but rather as a separate entity, whose empathic responsiveness allows the client to feel more "real." The idea of being recognized as a person in one's own right, and not just as an extension of another's hopes, wants, beliefs, and needs, can be empowering for the client. The energy released in this mutual recognition has the potential to nourish the client's desire to explore and develop other relationships.

Lara's case: empathy in action

Lara, a 27-year-old Albanian woman, had seen many social workers before coming to the community mental health center where I practiced. During her adolescence Lara suffered from major depression and was hospitalized after a suicide attempt. She had low self-esteem and few friends, and tended to isolate. She considered herself unattractive and believed she had nothing of interest to offer anyone. Having come to the United States from Albania at age six, Lara entered school unfamiliar with the English language. Consequently, she had difficulty reading and was placed in a special education class.

During her adolescence Lara was overweight and was teased by her peers. She avoided people because she felt "stupid and ugly" and felt she had "nothing to say." I let Lara know that I understood her feelings of worthlessness and shame, and the pain of her isolation. I felt sad for her.

From the painful life experiences and feelings Lara shared with me I understood why she felt uncomfortable with others. However, I experienced her very differently than she experienced herself. I said, "You come across to me as a caring person who gives a lot of herself to others. I believe that people would appreciate your sincerity and kindness as much as I do when they get to know you better." I wanted Lara to see and appreciate the impact she had made on me. It was important for Lara to know that she mattered, particularly since she had felt excluded and humiliated for much of her childhood and young adult years. The experience of "mattering," of having an impact on the other person, increases one's sense of relational competence. Lara became tearful and said that my understanding and caring meant a great deal to her.

Lara's story led me to recall some of my own adolescent memories of not feeling accepted by the "in" group, which made it easier for me to understand her pain. Being new to my neighborhood during my adolescent years also placed me on the "outside." Although I did not share Lara's exact experiences, I could put myself in her place, re-experience her loneliness, and demonstrate an understanding of her situation, and that I was authentically moved by the power of her feelings. My ability to resonate with her on a deep level helped us to create a mutually empathic connection. Over time, Lara began to feel more comfortable with herself and others. She slowly reached out to old friends and current acquaintances in an attempt to make new connections and reduce her self-imposed isolation.

A core feature of Benjamin's (1998) framework is the notion that any similarity between two people coexists in an uneasy balance with their inherent differences— cultural, psychological, biological, and sociological. Empathy, therefore, involves the worker's continuous efforts to fine-tune his/her understanding of the client in order to "get it right." Benjamin believes that when the client exerts a sense of agency and can see the clinician as a whole person, and when the clinician can see the client as a whole person, the empathic encounter becomes truly alive. Although Lara and I came from different cultural worldviews, the mutual empathy that marked the helping process helped bridge our different backgrounds.

Empathy and empowerment: Yvette's story

Since connections are important for self-definition and a sense of empowerment, creating the conditions that help others to use relational ties in constructive ways becomes a primary agenda for the practitioner. The following case vignette illustrates how as a social worker I used myself in a way that helped sensitize the client to the need to be empathic to others in her social environment. My relational orientation to practice fostered growth-promoting relationships on various levels—in the family, with the social worker in the mental health system, and with the caseworker in the child welfare system.

Yvette, a 36-year-old African-American woman diagnosed with schizophrenia, was referred to a court-affiliated mental health clinic in a large northern city by her probation officer. Yvette had a history of auditory hallucinations, for which she had been prescribed psychotropic medication. Prior to commencing treatment, she terminated a long-term relationship with the father of her twin daughters, aged two and a half. During this period she had stopped taking her medication, which resulted in her screaming and crying uncontrollably while her children were at home. A neighbor called the police who took her to a hospital where she was admitted to the psychiatric unit. Her children were placed with a local child welfare agency while she was hospitalized. Pursuant to her discharge treatment plan, Yvette came to see me weekly at a local mental health center in addition to seeing a psychiatrist for medication.

When Yvette began counseling, her twins had been in foster care for two months. The focus of her treatment was twofold: (1) compliance with her mediation regimen; and (2) working with the child welfare agency to have her daughters returned to her. Initially, Yvette reported that her caseworker from the agency was cold, unfeeling, and "not on my side." She blamed the agency and "the system" for taking her children away from her. After four months of taking her medication on a regular basis, Yvette's auditory hallucinations had considerably abated. She felt "ready to take care of her kids again" and was furious that the caseworker "wasn't helping her to get them back." She didn't believe the worker was doing her job properly nor did she think the child welfare worker cared about her or her children. Yvette wanted to call the caseworker's supervisor, contact the media, and "expose the system."

The worker encouraged Yvette to express her feelings in an appropriate manner, and empathized with her about her feelings of loss, rejection, and abandonment resulting from her romantic break-up and the loss of her children whom she loved dearly. After I had been seeing Yvette for about two months I said: "I think that if you want your children returned, you need to understand the role and responsibilities of your caseworker, her concerns, and what she expects from you." At first Yvette appeared not to understand and seemed a bit confused: "Why do I have to understand that bitch?" she said, rhetorically. I responded, "Regardless of how you feel about her personally, you are intelligent enough to understand that the child welfare caseworker is the key to getting your kids back. Her recommendation carries a lot of weight, and unless she feels you are ready, it won't happen for a long time." I added, "I know you are upset, but I really want to try to help you get your daughters back. I would like you to just think about what I've said, and we'll continue to discuss this." In the interim, Yvette continued to visit her twins regularly.

During my next session with Yvette, I explained the role and responsibilities of the agency caseworker and emphasized the fact that if the agency returned the children to Yvette and they were harmed, the agency and the worker would be held responsible. I asked, "Do you think the worker wants her name in the newspaper if something happens to the kids she is supervising?" Yvette was quiet for a while and then said, "No, I guess not." I continued, "Do you realize that the caseworker could lose her job, and that she probably needs a job as much as you need yours?" Yvette was silent as she thought this over. In the next few sessions, I continued to explore Yvette's interactions with her child welfare worker. We even did some role playing together. Yvette reported that the caseworker had become increasingly friendly and more sympathetic to her, and that she was taken her medication regularly, and that the auditory hallucinations had all but ceased. In December 2006 the children were returned to Yvette under supervision.

The ability of the client to be empathic toward the worker shows his or her capacity and willingness to appreciate another person. Being empathic does not mean that the client necessarily identifies with the worker's personal concerns. Rather, recognizing that worker and client can be moved by similar feelings creates a shared experience, which then helps them construct a sense of commonality (Jordan, 1983).

This capacity to recognize the other not merely as an object, but rather as a subject is an important part of early development and life-long growth. Intersubjectivity and mutuality begin with the mother–child relationship. When it may be appropriate for the dependent infant to see the mother solely as a gratifying object, the relationship must eventually become more mutual if the child is to develop into a healthy adult. Winnicott (1965) terms this the use of the object, when the infant perceives the mother figure as not just a projection, but as an external reality, with her own wants and needs. As the child matures, the parent not only influences the child, the child also influences the parent. A parallel process takes place in the social work relationship.

The Stone Center approach to empathy

The power and value of empathy are highlighted in constructing a feminist relational paradigm for practice. Building upon the work of selfobject/relational theorists such as Kohut and Winnicott, feminist theorists and practitioners from the Stone Center in Wellesley, Massachusetts, place the concept of empathy squarely at the center of human development (Jordan, 1989; Surrey et al., 1990). They consider the worker's use of empathy essential in relationship building. As demonstrated by the case of Lara, empathy provides a secure and safe context that maximizes the client's ability to feel free to be his/her authentic self. Stone Center scholars view empathy as a primary force that drives growth and development. Typically, it begins with mothers developing the capacity for empathy in their daughters through the process of same-sex role identification. Surrey et al. (1990) stress that, in most cultures, women live out their lives centered on the preparation for, and exercise of, a care-taking role. Early and continuous sex-role identification with a female figure reinforced by gender-specific socialization processes foster the capacity of females to be attuned to others (Chodorow, 1978). While both males and females are able to recognize and label the affective experience of another person (i.e. display cognitive awareness), Chodorow believes that females have been socialized to demonstrate a greater degree of responsiveness to others while most men have not been socialize to connect in quite the same way. Eisenberg & Strayer (1987) have conducted studies showing that gender differences develop because males and females are socialized differently. Similarly, Gilligan (1982) contends that girls and boys experience different paths of socialization, with girls being taught an ethic of caring rather than an ethic of justice. The difference becomes even more obvious in adolescence, when males are taught to "act out" (i.e. hide) their feelings when vulnerable (Hoffman, 1997).

Boundary management: balancing self-autonomy with affective connection

Stone Center theorist Judith Jordan (1983, p. 13) views empathy as:

> An ability that requires a complex integration of cognitive and emotional capacities that provide a foundation for human connection ... The affective component comprises feelings of emotional connectedness, a capacity to fully take in and contain the feelings of the other person. The cognitive component rests on one's integral sense of self and the capacity to act on the basis of that sense of self.

Jordan (1984) adds another dimension, stressing that empathy requires a complex integration of balancing cognitive and emotional capacities, providing the basic foundation of human connection. She suggests that empathy can be emotional *and* rational, affective and intellectual, and that the two can mutually co-exist. The challenge for the clinician is to empathize on an emotional level while exercising cognitive capacities needed to distinguish those feelings induced by the client as opposed to those feelings engendered by personal experience.

Belenky and her colleagues (1986) see the capacity for empathy, which they call "connected knowing," as a way of thinking and feeling. They believe that since ideas come from experience, the only way to truly understand the other person's ideas is to attempt to understand the experience that led to their formation. This requires putting oneself in the place of the other and seeing the world from the other's perspective.

Connected knowing implies that empathy emerges through care, and caring represents a quest for understanding. People can only approximate another person's point of view, which requires that social workers ask questions in order to learn about their client's culture, background, and the world in which they live (Belenky et al., 1986). Feedback from clients is the only way in which practitioners can be fully in tune with the client and be able to adjust their perceptions accordingly. It is important to take risks, be genuine, be respectful, and be able to acknowledge when you are not being effectively empathic. You will know this if you reach for client feedback and if you are keenly tuned into verbal and non-verbal cues. The deeper and more trusting the client–worker relationship, the more the client reveals, and the easier it is for the practitioner to see the world through the client's eyes.

Empathy requires a high level of cognitive structuring on the part of the social worker, who must simultaneously balance his/her own perception of reality with the meaning the client makes of a given situation. This requires an ability to oscillate from observer to participant, allowing the worker to "be" with the client without losing a sense of his/her own affective experiences. Oscillation between focusing on the self and focusing on the other takes skill, keen self-awareness, concentration, and boundary flexibility. It is this free flow of energy that is required for a true empathic exchange to occur.

Elements of emotional attunement and connected knowing coexist in every empathic encounter. Balancing affect and cognition is not always easy. For example, if the social worker and the client share the same experience or have a similar life history, over-identification may become an issue and a blurring of the boundaries might take place. When there is a momentary over-identification between the clinician and client, the relational social worker rapidly shifts attention from the self to the client continuing to differentiate self from the other simultaneously and on an ongoing basis. In order to accomplish this level of mutuality, the worker must be grounded enough so as not to encourage closeness in order to gratify his or her own needs, or become too distant out of the fear of merger (Jordan, 1984).

Being able to feel deeply with another person suggests that one is able to temporarily suspend ego boundaries without fear of losing oneself in the process. Contrary to past psychoanalytic notions wherein workers were overly concerned about maintaining emotional distance out of fear of encountering their own countertransference reactions, the "relational" worker experiences and willingly expresses a wide range of thoughts and feelings, facilitating a sense of emotional connection with the client. Feeling deeply with another does not necessarily imply a form of "regressive merging," nor does it suggest a "blurring of the self." Rather, empathy is a sophisticated cognitive and emotional activity in which one person is able to experience the thoughts and feelings of another person as if they were one's own, while simultaneously being aware of the difference (Jordan, 1984). These ideas imply that the worker is mature and capable of maintaining a relatively clear sense of self and flexible ego boundaries to allow for the high degree of emotional and cognitive integration essential for empathy to be effective.

The power and value of empathic communication have been consistently recognized in social work literature as a tool used to enhance the helping relationship. Developing the capacity for empathy is a developmental goal, a dynamic part of the helping process, and a principal lever for change. In the Stone Center paradigm, the emphasis is placed on mutual empathy, which involves mutual participation and mutual action.

Feminist relational practitioners who strive to be authentic are active and expressive in their use of themselves. It is this critical ability to elaborate on one's own feelings and thoughts in the presence of another that allows for real engagement. Communication takes place through body language, facial expressions, affect, intonation, and reflection of manifest and latent content. When the worker responds in a genuinely empathic way, it is a kind of self-disclosure in which reactions are shared in the presence of the client. Distinct from the traditional approach, mutual empathy involves a conceptual shift—from a uni-directional technique in which the worker shows genuine concern, to bi-directional movement in which worker and client feel each other's active involvement and are engaged in genuine sharing.

Mutual empathy: Leslie's case

The following case of Leslie illustrates my attempt to establish a mutually empathic relationship with a 17-year-old adolescent (who was mentioned in Chapter 3). As she approached her senior year in high school, Leslie increasingly expressed confusion and fear about going on to college. Shuttling back and forth between her divorced parents—one in Colorado and one in New York—she had lacked a stable home base for many years. For the past three years she had been living with her father and made a relatively good adjustment to her new town. It was not surprising that leaving home again would be difficult for her. Having to make the decision about whether she was ready for college, and if, so which college to attend, framed an identity crisis for Leslie that was similar to what most teens go through: Who am I? What do I want? Where do I belong? Will I make friends?

With my help, Leslie and her father researched different colleges and Leslie applied to several in the Midwest and Northeast. One day she proudly announced that she was accepted into two of them—a private college, her first choice, as well as an excellent state university. I was very excited for Leslie and had a big smile on my face when I said, "I am so thrilled for you, that is great news, Leslie. What an accomplishment for you!" It was important that she really *feel* my happiness, since this moment was one of the most positive, life-affirming experiences Leslie had had in her recent past. When I asked her which school she was considering, she stated that although she was really happy to get accepted into both, she did not think her dad could afford the private college. Sensitive to her father's financial situation, Leslie said, "It would place an enormous burden on him, so I decided to accept the state university's offer. It's also closer to home."

At our next meeting, Leslie was able to share that not only was she disappointed about not going to the college she wanted most, but she also felt sad about not applying to the school near where her mother lived—her original intention. Having talked with her mother on the phone a few months earlier, Leslie realized that her mom was neither sober nor stable. Leslie told me, "I don't think I'm ready to deal with her. It's best for me not to see or even talk to her at this point." She cried when I said that it must have been painful for her to accept the fact that her dreams of going back home to her family and friends were shattered. By creating an environment marked by validation and empathic attunement, I was providing Leslie with a place where she could feel respected and be herself.

I was impressed with Leslie's growing sense of maturity and her ability to understand some of the realities upon which she based her decision and told her so: "Wow, I am really impressed with how much thought you have put into this decision and how mature you are being right now. I know you are disappointed in giving up your dream school, but the state university is excellent and a great choice. I am really proud of you," I said. Leslie clearly felt my excitement and my pride in her accomplishments. She beamed and said that for the first time she experienced a sense of someone actually cared about what she wanted instead of using her as a pawn for their own needs (referring to her parents).

Empathy is a quality that can lead to more fulfilling relationships. An emotionally healthy infant "tunes into" the mother's state of mind, not just to her behaviors (Beebe & Lachmann, 2002). As one matures, the ability to empathize on a higher level is one indicator of a healthy, integrated ego. Modeling this for the client does not necessarily mean disclosing personal information; rather, the worker is moved by the client's experience and responds accordingly. The client, in response, feels the worker's response, and knows that he or she has made an impact. In Leslie's situation I shared that I too had attended a state university instead of a private one of my choice for financial reasons, and thought that I got a great education and made wonderful friends. With adolescents, the moment of mutual empathy often comes when you are genuine and "real" with them.

It is important to underscore that in the empathic exchange, the worker must truly experience the client's affective state in order to make an impact. In relational–cultural terms, this ability to deeply feel "with" the other person is called *affective resonance*. Affective resonance is a form of physiological arousal in which the worker experiences a vicarious emotional response while cognitively aware that the source of the feeling originates from the other person (Jordan, 1997a). The idea is for the client to feel that he/she has moved you, to know that there was an impact on you, and vice versa. The worker sometimes taps into memories of a similar situation of his/her own in order to intensify the connection, shifting back and forth between the worker's and the client's cognitive and affective processes. If successful, the empathic process is validating and deepens the sense of engagement between client and worker.

In working with Leslie, it was particularly easy for me to communicate to her that she mattered and to join in her sadness. In light of the fact that Leslie did not have a secure or stable mother figure, I felt particularly nurturing toward her. Furthermore, my ability to relate to her affective and cognitive state was deepened by the fact that she possessed qualities that I genuinely admired and could relate to—a natural "earthy style," sensible values, and an interest in books and music of my generation.

Mutual empathy should not be confused with over-identification or countertransference. Clearly, each person in the client–worker relationship has a different role and status, which serves to protect boundary integrity while allowing worker and client to feel connected to one another. According to Surrey et al. (1990, p. 1), "Mutual empathy is not so much a matter of reciprocity—I give to you and then you give to me—but rather a quality of relatedness, movement, a dynamic of relationship."

While there may be a momentary surrender of feelings following affective cues, the clinician should always maintain an awareness of the source of the feeling. Because, according to relational theory, movement and change happen through a matrix of connection, disconnection, and re-connection, the worker needs to be in touch with a vast array of thoughts and feelings that are in direct response to what the client is experiencing. Misunderstandings and differences, as well as connections and similarities that arise in the mutual flow, have to be negotiated and accepted for what they are in order for both the client and worker to grow (Surrey et al., 1990).

On the cultural and political side

The feminist-oriented relational approach has expanded its theoretical framework to include a heightened awareness of the diverse cultural and socio-political contexts that shape growth and development and relational experiences—what the Stone Center scholars refer to as a "relational–cultural" approach to practice. The willingness to be genuinely empathic to another's worldview can provide a basis for a more collaborative relationship, one in which both worker and client can learn from their differences as well as from their similarities. Thus, cross-cultural empathy can help to deepen one's understanding of the client as well as to enhance a sense of mutuality.

This approach is based on the belief that any empathic connection cannot be fully realized without great sensitivity to the socio-cultural context in which the client is embedded. Gender-related experiences intersect with socioeconomic status, race, age, ethnic, sexual orientation, and other forms of difference that situate people in a socially stratified society which then become powerful determinants of the reality of their lives (Jordan et al., 2004). Thus, if empathic communication is to be successful, it is critical that the worker understand that the client's worldview is filtered through a specific cultural frame of reference, including power differentials that exist across racial, ethnic, and gender lines.

The client's perception of power, or lack of power, has been identified as a critical ingredient in the worker's ability to establish a cross-cultural complementary helping relationship (Dyche & Zayas, 2001; Pinderhughes, 1979). Openly acknowledging the impact of cultural forces and power differentials is important, especially if the worker is part of a dominant group that the client sees as the oppressor. This can bring about emotional discomfort, but it is necessary to validate the other person's experience; failure to validate the client's perception and experience with others when crossing racial, ethnic, or class lines can contribute to further disconnections with the worker. Knowing that resources and opportunities are often rewarded or withheld based on cultural privilege, it becomes important to bring power differentials and cultural determinants to the surface in an attempt to connect empathically with clients (Surrey et al., 1990). The following case of Joan illustrates the significance of socio-cultural issues.

Joan, a 45-year-old Afro-Caribbean woman with whom I worked for two years, is a good example of someone whose sense of empowerment increased in the context of a clinician–client relationship that was marked by cultural sensitivity, mutual empathy, and mutual respect. Joan had been a successful high-level bank executive for the past 12 years. However, she had recently been subjected to daily criticism from the newly appointed bank president, a Caucasian male, who was connected to the "old boys' network" in the banking community. His insidious and constant belittling led her to believe that she was incompetent and that she had no course but to leave her job. This kind of emotional abuse eroded Joan's self-esteem to the point that when she sought help, she stated that her "world was falling apart."

Joan had dealt with discrimination previously at the workplace but did not expect it at this point in her career. We spent weeks exploring her feelings of shame, disappointment, and anger. I was deeply moved by, and open to, Joan's pain. As a female professional, this resonated with experiences I have had in my own life and although I recognized the differences, I shared this with Joan. Joan saw that she had made an impact on me. I related that I felt sad that she was unable to maintain a positive self-image because of the discriminatory actions of her boss. And so she was left feeling helpless in the face of an oppressive force that she could not control.

When Joan discussed her work, she presented as articulate, bright, and clearly very competent. I was genuinely impressed with Joan's knowledge and skills and communicated my confidence in her by telling her this. I also reminded her that her sense of powerlessness and disconnection was exacerbated by the fact that she was culturally and socially isolated, since she was the only minority female bank executive at her workplace. Joan began to develop a heightened awareness of the social and political forces at play. A period of self-reflection unfolded, and she was able to explore alternative career opportunities. Eventually, Joan found another job in a work environment that was more compatible with her strengths and needs.

This kind of empathic connection established between worker and client can provide a blueprint that fosters the client's ability to form supportive, sustaining relationships beyond the helping one. Empathy can be viewed as the fuel or energy that drives the relational approach, and the client–worker relationship can be seen as the vehicle through which one experiences a basic sense of connection. An enhanced feeling of power can grow out of the healthy interaction with empathically attuned others contributing to the capacity to act in the environment with a greater sense of self-efficacy and purposefulness. Jean Baker Miller (1991b) calls this sense of being able to effect change in the larger relational context *agency-in-community*.

Social work best practices for developing empathic relationships

Social workers can strengthen empathic connections with clients through practicing a number of proven techniques:

- *Intentionally seek intense emotional attunement*: attempt to feel the person's emotions as if they were your own. Start where the client is, allowing yourself to be vulnerable and open. Be attuned to the client, feeling with and validating their affective states, thoughts, and perceptions.
- *Create a relational image*: identify a situation in your own life, similar to the clients when similar feelings arise.
- *Share with clients only what is necessary*: selectively inform clients of your reactions, thoughts, feelings. Allow yourself to be known in ways that give the client helpful feedback and can allow them to feel that s/he has made an impact on you.
- *Open yourself to being affected by the other*: be authentic. Your responses should be congruent with the client's thoughts and feelings. Be aware that as two people connect, the distinction between them may blur.
- *Model authentic empathic attunement*: rather than being a passive repository, you may provide a reparative opportunity for earlier disconnections in which parts of the self were invalidated.

In summary, empathy is more than just a technique; it is related to one's capacity for emotional connection. It allows for the existence of individual differences without the obliteration of individuality. Genuine empathy takes place in relational, cultural, economic, historical, and social contexts, and, hopefully, leads to an increase in the client's sense of well-being and sense of connectedness to others. The more connected clients feel to their social worker, the more they will open up and share information that the practitioner can use to develop an assessment and plan of intervention.

5 Assessment
A relational–cultural point of view

Since social work concerns itself with the person-in-environment as a way of understanding individuals and their problems, it is essential that a relational assessment include the context of family, friends, groups, community, the material and socioeconomic conditions that shape experience, the dimensions of identity, taking into consideration society's response to race, ethnicity, gender, sexual orientation, religion, disability, society's response to those elements, as well as the quality and quantity of relational connections (Smith et al., 2006).

Based on the relational–cultural model developed by Stone Center practitioner/theoreticians at Wellesley College, this chapter examines relational processes, the structural components of relationships, and the implications of chronic disconnection within the context of family, group, and community. In essence, relational thinking shapes the assessment process and possible points of intervention that flow from a relational viewpoint.

This chapter provides a relational–cultural framework which integrates relational theory, psychodynamic concepts, and feminist scholarship in the assessment process. It is important for clinicians to keep in mind that there is often a link between current problems and early relationships. Clients may not recognize the link between their own emotional state, behavior, current problems and circumstances, and the significance of relational factors, patterns, and interactions. Women, in particular, organize themselves in the context of important relationships and strive to maintain a sense of connectedness with others. Considerations that arise from the emotional presence or lack of presence of others form a basic component of one's self-experience (Silverstein et al., 2006). Thus, relationship variables are not just viewed as an "add-on"; they are central to health and key to a comprehensive assessment, planning, and treatment.

Assessment

Assessment is the heart of social work practice and the foundation upon which our thinking and doing is based. There are many different types of assessment: bio-psycho-social assessments, concrete needs assessments, mental status exams, family assessments, and community and organizational assessments. Levine (2002, p. 830) formulated a useful generic definition of assessment as "the process of systematically collecting data about a client's functioning and monitoring progress on an ongoing basis. [It is a] process of problem selection and specification that is guided in social work by a person-in-environment orientation."

Good assessments and the decisions that follow involve the abilities to: (1) amass and organize a variety of facts; (2) analyze the information together *with* the client; (3) understand the issues; and (4) determine the goals of the therapeutic process (Meyer, 1993). According to Germain and Gitterman (1996), assessment tasks common to most practice approaches include:

1   Collecting data on life stressors and their degree of severity; the perception of the stressor; internal and external resources available for coping; cultural, biological, psychological, cognitive, familial, and environmental factors; and strengths and limitations.
2   Organizing data in a way that reveals significant patterns and clarifies meaning.
3   Analyzing and synthesizing data in order to draw inferences about strengths and limitations, environmental resources and deficits, and level of client-environment fit.

Feminist scholars Miller and Stiver (1997) at the Wellesley College Center for Research on Women have identified five growth-fostering relational characteristics that are helpful both in making assessments and evaluating outcomes: (1) mutuality; (2) a sense of empowerment; (3) a sense of self-worth and self-esteem; (4) desire for more connection; and (5) the capacity to deal with inter-personal conflict. In addition, an evaluation of the client's capacities for engagement, authenticity, commitment, attunement, acceptance of diversity and difference, and mutual empathy can enhance the assessment and intervention process (Genero et al., 1992).

A relational assessment is broader and more inclusive than a bio-psycho-social assessment. It is a mutual, ongoing process that encourages clients' active participation in the collection of data and in thinking through the underlying forces and relational patterns that shape their experience. Clients are involved in the decision-making process to the fullest extent possible. This dynamic collaboration is used to enhance the clients' awareness of self and others, and to evaluate their social supports, relationships, or lack of relational connections and available resources. The social worker who thinks relationally listens for clients' strengths, resources, and capacities, trying to find ways to capitalize on them. Sometimes this means helping clients to improve the quality of their relationships, to encourage new connections, or to help them extricate themselves from destructive relationships.

An effective relational assessment emphasizes relational connections—linkages as well as disconnections—not only for information and evaluation purposes, but also as a primary target for intervention. It pays close attention to the quality and quantity of relational structures and processes that exist in the client's life space. In addition, an evaluation of the client's capacities for engagement, authenticity, commitment, attunement, acceptance of diversity and difference, and mutual empathy can enhance the assessment and intervention process (Genero et al., 1992).

It is important to note that in the assessment process attention is paid to all relationships, past and present, across the client's life span. Individuals who are not physically present in the client's life are sometimes more significant than those who are physically present. Often, it is the relationship that the client does not talk about, or that carries the most anger and pain, which is most significant in the healing process. These "disconnects" become targeted areas for assessment and intervention. Thus, the visible (or sometimes invisible) thread of relational ties and connections, or lack of connection to individuals, community, and social supports are important factors in assessment and intervention approaches. For example, the refusal of a child in foster care to visit with his or her mother may be an indication that his/her reluctance is not necessarily a rejection of the mother, but a manifestation of the painful reminder of the absence of her/his mother. The exploration of this disconnection may be the key point at which the social worker intervenes.

A relational assessment does not preclude bio-psycho-social factors and attention to internal or intrapsychic issues in people's lives; rather it enhances the dimensions of a bio-psycho-social assessment. Especially significant are the ways in which clients believe others view them; these images are acquired through repeated transactions with others and are referred to as relational images. The feelings induced in the clinician as a result of what transpires between the client and worker in the treatment process is often a barometer of what the client is feeling and experiencing.

A relational perspective uses what clients share about their lives, and both rework the story together so that it has meaning to the client (Goldstein et al., 2009). In telling the "story," the worker asks questions that prompt the client to talk about the important people in his or her life, and attempts to ascertain the quality as well as quantity of relationships. Research has shown that it is the quality of the relationship that is more important than the quantity (Liang et al., 1998).

The focal aspects of a relational assessment include

- current life situation, especially the quality and nature of interpersonal relationships, and the significance they have to the client;
- history, family background, and relational themes and patterns in the way family members relate to each other, and how these patterns are carried over into other significant relationships;
- quality of early caretaking and interpersonal experiences surrounding transactions between worker and client; and
- gender, cultural, sexual orientation, and other environmental factors.

The following case will illustrate how the clinician can draw on relational thinking in developing an assessment of the client and his/her situation. In particular, it illustrates the importance of the effect of the quality of relationships in one's family of origin as well as the current relationship with a significant life partner on one's ability to function successfully in the role of a new parent. In this role many adjustments have to be made on an emotional and physical level in order to bond with one's infant. The father's ability to be supportive of the mother through pregnancy and childbirth has been shown to be highly predictive of the mother's postpartum adjustment (Howell, 1981).

Presentation of problem/history

Jennifer is a 37-year-old female of Hispanic/European descent. She is a registered nurse who has been working in a critical care unit in a local hospital for the past ten years, where she is well liked and respected. She has been divorced for two years and is living by herself in an apartment near her former boyfriend, Glen, who has custody of their now 18-month-old son Jonathan. Jennifer had been seen jointly with her ex-husband by the worker, who received a call from Jennifer two years later, stating that she wanted to see the clinician again, this time by herself. Jennifer briefly explained that shortly after her divorce, she entered into a relationship with Glen, and became pregnant. She went on to say that she had recently been released from jail, having been imprisoned for six months on a felony assault charge.

History of problem

After a five-year marriage, Jennifer's husband said he "wanted out." He gave no concrete reason, but Jennifer felt he had never really been emotionally available. Two years after the divorce, she entered into a relationship with Glen and became pregnant. After the birth, Jennifer became very depressed. She reported to her doctor, boyfriend, and pediatrician that she had visions of hurting Jonathan and had thoughts of throwing him out the window. A visit to the ER resulted in a brief hospitalization. She was placed on medication and discharged but continued to have thoughts and feelings consistent with a diagnosis of postpartum major depressive disorder with brief psychotic episodes. One such episode, during which she tried to smother Jonathan—an attempt to stop his crying—resulted in her boyfriend calling 911, her subsequent arrest, placement in a psychiatric hospital, and incarceration for six months. Upon release, she was placed on probation, continued with her medication regimen, and mandated to attend therapy.

Family background/personal history

The oldest of three children, Jennifer was raised by two parents in a small Northeastern city. Not much is known about her brothers other than the older one is mentally ill and estranged from Jennifer, and the younger one is single, lives nearby, and is more present in Jennifer's life now. Originally, her parents, now deceased, were from Peru. Her mother was indigenous to the area, and her father was of German/Spanish heritage, having moved there from Spain. While in Peru her father had two children with another woman before meeting Jennifer's mother.

Jennifer stated that she is not strongly identified with her Hispanic heritage. Growing up, she was cut off from her extended family, most of whom remained in Peru. Once in America, her family was determined to acculturate, and did not maintain familial and communal networks in Peru or with the Latin American community in the new country. All of the men with whom she has had serious relationships were Anglo.

Jennifer's father was distant, controlling, and continuously belittled her mother. Her mom was passive, and could not protect herself or Jennifer from her father's "bullying." Jennifer's father's tyrannical behavior prevented her from developing friendships throughout her childhood years.

When Jennifer was 17 her mother became ill with breast cancer, and Jennifer had to leave school to care for her. After her mother died, Jennifer's father abandoned Jennifer and her brothers to return to Peru to his other family. Jennifer became the surrogate parent for her siblings. She was left to pay the bills, handle the funeral arrangements, and mourn her mother's death—alone. Having learned that her father died while she was in prison, it was only then that she was able to get in touch with her anger toward him for abandoning her and her brothers. Jennifer eventually got her GED and went on to nursing school to obtain her RN.

Current situation

At the time Jennifer reinitiated treatment, she had not had contact with Jonathan from the time he was 6 months until he was 15 months. Currently, she has supervised visitation and spends about two days a week with him and some weekends. She is back at her current job where she is working in an administrative capacity closely supervised by management. She has a network of friends at work—mainly other nurses—with whom she has positive relationships and who are a source of emotional support. They are a culturally diverse group who offer her advice on various ways to parent Jonathan—often contradictory and at odds with her own instincts.

When Jennifer re-entered therapy, she was somewhat guarded and stated that she was fearful of exploring her painful past. But as therapy progressed, she was able to put her trust in the clinician who could provide her with the right holding environment for repair and compensation. Gradually, she was able to talk about her feelings, the recent trauma in her life, as well as her mother's death and her father's abandonment..

But right from the beginning she *was* open to talking about her son. She told the clinician that she had been overwhelmed taking care of a helpless infant, not feeling she "had what it took" to give him what he needed. Nor did she feel the support of her boyfriend. She had no mother, father, or close family members to help her, nurture her, or give her advice. Having a baby made her long for her own mother, who Jennifer had idealized, describing her as a "saint." When Jonathan cried she could not comfort him, and there was no one to comfort her. Now, she was in the position of having to be a mother, crying out for help herself.

As therapy progressed, Jennifer became increasingly open to talking about how she felt about herself as a mother, acknowledging she was "never really present" for Jonathan. Her own depression was a heavy burden to bear. After a few months, Jonathan and his father joined Jennifer for a session. During the visit, Jonathan repeatedly returned to the clinician to be picked up instead of his mother. Jennifer said that it was painful to observe Jonathan's preference for the therapist.

Jennifer's relationship with Glen, who by this time had partnered with another woman, had grown tense. Jennifer recognized that he used his custody of Jonathan to assume total control of their son. She felt disconnected from both Glen and Jonathan, but wanted desperately to resume her maternal role. Not only did she long to establish a bond with Jonathan, but her ensuing loneliness and psychological distress was exacerbated by Glen's rejection of her.

Although Jennifer focused on building a relationship with her son, she did not have the necessary relational tools, family supports, or parenting skills. Her therapist recognized that Jennifer needed some help in learning how to relate to her baby. She also recognized that she needed a supportive network of friends and family. Jennifer's trust in the worker deepened as the clinician provided her with the right holding environment for repair and compensation, and begin to explore her painful past. Although fearful, Jennifer was gradually able to get in touch with her long repressed feelings of resentment for both mother and dad—her mother for dying so young, and her dad for his abandonment and emotional abuse of her mother. Gradually, she came to see her mother more realistically, to mourn her, and to confront her father's emotional abuse and abandonment.

Relational assessment

Jennifer did not receive adequate nurturing from her mother, who was emotionally dependent on Jennifer, seeking the warmth and support she did not get from her husband. Mom's dependency on Jennifer was intensified by her illness, just when Jennifer's primary developmental task was individuating from her family of origin while, at the same time, maintaining a secure relationship with them. According to the work of the Stone Center, psychological growth is viewed as a relational process which is based on differentiation and elaboration rather than disengagement and separation (Jordan, 1985). Unfortunately, Jennifer's family system was not one in which she could feel a secure connection. Due to family responsibilities, relational ties with peers were attenuated as well.

Clearly, Jennifer did not have "good enough" relationships with others. Her connections for the most part lacked emotional responsiveness, mutual empathy, mutual empowerment, authenticity, and cultural similarity. Jennifer's sense of self-worth, competence, and motivation to connect with other people was damaged. Incarceration further exacerbated her shame, guilt, self-blame, and sense of being marginalized, resulting in further disconnection from others.

Jennifer had over-identified with Jonathan as a helpless, vulnerable infant whom she could not protect, as she herself had not been protected. Her attempt to extinguish his life was a way to eradicate her own pain. Jennifer's illness, postpartum depression with psychosis—a disorder which blurs the boundaries between the person and others around them—was not properly diagnosed by her doctors.

According to Daniel Hall-Favin (2012), a leading expert on the symptoms of postpartum depression, if left untreated for a few months or longer, it can lead to postpartum psychosis, including symptoms of hallucinations and delusions, confusion and disorientation, and attempts to harm oneself or one's baby. In addition to hormonal changes, one of the causes of this condition is a lack of support from a partner or loved one.

Jennifer's most significant relationship at the time of Jonathan's birth was with Glen. But he turned out to be as cold, distant, and controlling as her father had been, leaving Jennifer feeling unsupported. Her closest friends had been the other nurses at work, but she was cut off from them when she took a leave to assume her new parental role. Her depression left her unable to form a consistent and gratifying attachment with her son.

She was incapable of giving emotional sustenance to this helpless, demanding infant at a time in her life when she herself was not receiving adequate emotional support. The therapist recognized that Jennifer needed a supportive network of friends and family.

Mutual participation in relationships is an essential part of relational functioning and development. The Mutual Psychological Development Questionnaire (MPDQ) developed by Genero et al. (1992) is a standardized instrument based on a relational framework of psychological development described by Miller (1986) and Jordan (1985). See Appendix A of this book for a complete scale and description of this instrument. Jennifer's responses on the MPDQ scale suggests that her relationship with Glen—her most intimate relationship—ranked low on the six elements of mutuality identified as follows: empathy, engagement, authenticity, empowerment, zest, and diversity. This lack of mutuality is associated with low self-esteem, a lack of emotional availability, and can affect feelings of shame, anger, and depression.

Treatment plan/goals

Jennifer's primary treatment goal was to establish a mutually loving relationship with her son. However, the clinician knew that this would be difficult. Jonathan was at a critical age when the separation from Jennifer occurred. Jennifer needed to develop more confidence in herself as a parent, and to gain the skills and tools that would allow her to achieve a secure attachment with her son.

Jennifer's treatment plans and goals included:

- The development of a mutual loving and secure relationship with her son.
- The ability to become attuned to her son's needs so as to develop and strengthen a mutual attachment with each other.
- The development of a sense of confidence in her mothering abilities and trust in her own maternal instincts.
- The ability to use the client–worker relationship in a way that would help her to trust others again and to feel secure; to validate herself as a caring mother; and to provide "mirroring" in Kohut's terms, to confirm her sense of self as a worthwhile and whole person.
- The ability to use the client–worker relationship in a way that would develop a sense of mutual empathy and empowerment that she could transfer to other relationships.
- Decreasing her depression and increasing her sense of energy and motivation to connect to others.
- The development of a productive, working relationship with her psychiatrist, the child welfare worker, and a child-focused infant–mother psychologist with the goal of developing a support network of caring professionals working toward increasing visitation with her son and stabilizing her mental health.
- The development of a support network of friends, co-workers, and family; in particular her brother, who was her closest relative.

The paradox of connection in a relational–cultural context

The feminist relational assessment approach to social work practice is embedded in a cultural context. Issues such as gender, power, domination, and subordination impact on client self-determination, access to institutional resources, and available opportunities for healthy connections. In the relational school of thought, the action of having power *over* is replaced by the idea of power *with*. The *power with*, or mutual power model, makes the development of empowering relationships central. Power *with* others connotes that each person is empowered through the relationship. The relationship then works to sustain mutual empathy and interest, which does not involve winning or losing but rather a commitment to deepen the connection (Surrey, 1987).

A sense of empowerment can come from both innate strengths and environmental resources and supports. Individuals with a positive self-image and adequate self-esteem are more likely to have the energy and motivation to take action in their environment. Concurrently, the environment must provide the opportunities, concrete resources, and social supports that will allow clients to actualize their potentials and sense of empowerment. The relational worker focuses on the space in between—that context in which the interaction takes place.

A number of relational characteristics foster growth: (1) mutuality; (2) feeling empowered to take action; (3) gaining a greater sense of self-worth and validation; (4) an increased desire for more connection; and (5) the capacity to deal with conflict (Jordan, 1997b; Miller & Stiver, 1997). A healthy sense of connection to others, in which the client feels truly listened to, understood, and respected, is an important source of empowerment. As suggested by Nancy Chodorow (1978), a sense of connection to others is *the* central organizing feature in women's development.

Culturally, it is generally more acceptable for females to seek out relationships and to stay connected longer and more intensely than males. The importance of social supports and relationships in women's health and adjustment has been well documented. Although there is a range of capacities for relationship among men as well as women, the research has supported what I have found in my own practice—that most males have more tenuous relational ties than most females, especially when it comes to friendships (Kimmel, 2004). The challenge for the social worker is to help boys and men recognize the value of intimacy, and to encourage them to discover relational strategies for reaching out to others in authentic and growth-producing ways.

A brief case vignette demonstrates how I used the relational–cultural perspective as a way to develop an assessment of Tom, a 42-year-old Caucasian male who was caught in what Miller and Stiver (1997, p. 81) have termed the "central relational paradox." This central paradox refers to a longing for affirming relationships, while the fear of connection keeps one from revealing his or her most vulnerable parts, thereby preventing true connection. This paradox had special relevance for Tom, a middle-aged man who desired connection, but due to his image of masculinity as tough and cool, was unable to acknowledge his need for validating relationships.

I met with Tom and his wife Betty for marriage counseling for several months. Tom struggled to make a living as a construction worker. He was a skilled, experienced laborer who spent long, hard hours at work. Yet he had not received a pay raise in the last two years, nor did he have the confidence to ask for one. His wife was dissatisfied because he did not make enough money for them to live comfortably. This hurt his pride, especially since other men he knew in their suburban community were better able to provide for their families. He felt a sense of humiliation at not being able to support his family in the lifestyle his wife was accustomed to before their marriage.

Betty accused Tom of being an alcoholic, a charge that he denied. She was convinced that his drinking would destroy Tom, their marriage, and their family, which included two small children, 7-year-old Johnny and 9-year-old Mary. Tom was often explosive at home. He had a particularly difficult relationship with Johnny, with whom he was punitive and critical. Johnny was scared of his father's outbursts and Betty tried to protect him from her husband as best as she could. Betty's constant criticism of Tom and Tom's poor parenting skills only added to his sense of isolation and failure.

In addition to feeling like an outsider with his wife and children in his own home, Tom was distant from his family of origin. He saw his parents occasionally but did not feel close to them, and he had virtually no relationship with his sister who lived in the Southwest. Weekends were usually spent with his mother-in-law with whom he had a hostile relationship. When his wife brought up the fact that Tom was adopted in one of our sessions, he said, "It doesn't matter and I don't want to talk about it." He was very firm about this. At about this time in our work together, Betty decided to stop attending sessions, and I continued to see Tom alone.

I believed Tom wanted to continue to see me in part because we had a good working relationship in addition to the fact that he had no one with whom he could talk comfortably. I commented that it did not seem as if he was connected with anyone in his life who made him feel good about himself. When I asked Tom if he had any friends with whom he enjoyed spending time, he simply said "no."

However, he did mention that he used to "shoot hoops" with a buddy from high school but had not seen him in about five years. They just lost touch and had gone their separate ways. When I brought up the idea of reconnecting with his friend he was reluctant to do so. Alienated from his family and friends, the only real connection he had was to his alcohol. In his struggle to shut out pain and disappointment he retreated into his own world, numbing his own feelings and becoming oblivious to the feelings of others.

Looking at this case from a relational point of view, I realized that Tom lacked relational awareness and had few satisfying relationships except for the therapeutic one we had established together. According to Judith Jordan (2004, p. 54), "relational awareness is not about analyzing relationships; it involves an attitude of openness to learning about relational patterns." For Tom, being open and accessible to others was a sign of weakness. Uncertain of his own identity, ashamed of his economic plight in life, feeling excluded by his family, he was like an egg with a fragile shell, desperate to protect himself from shattering. Consequently, Tom allowed himself few meaningful interpersonal connections so as not to risk piercing his emotional barrier.

Tom, like other individuals who do not feel valued or powerful, would sometimes self-isolate; at other times, he displaced his anger and shame onto his family. Paradoxically speaking, Tom desired to be in relationships demonstrated by his commitment to his family. However, under stress, his strategy was to become aggressive or to disconnect. He would not permit himself to be vulnerable or to express his needs. Neither would he allow himself to explore his feelings and thoughts about his adoption. His disconnection from important parts of his history, such as the facts surrounding his adoption, led me to wonder how much intimacy he could really tolerate.

As in Tom's case, I believe that behind many individual problems lay chronic disconnections, violations, or distorted images of self and other. Sometimes the precipitating factors that create tension and maladaptive behaviors are rooted in environmental stress; most of the time they result from an interlocking of inner and outer forces. An important role for the social worker is to assist clients with establishing healthier and more trusting relationships that may result in more effective psycho-social functioning.

Jean Baker Miller and Irene Stiver (1997) identify five beneficial components—what they call "five good things"—that result from relationships characterized by empathy, honesty, and respect:

1 an increased sense of zest or well-being that comes with feeling connected to others;
2 the motivation to put feelings and thoughts into words and action;
3 increased knowledge about oneself and others;
4 an increased sense of self-worth; and
5 a desire for more connection.

The social worker who is knowledgeable about these "five good things" can help the client develop optimal relationships which can lead to a greater sense of self, the motivation to be a more active agent in the environment, and enhanced self-esteem—outcomes central to and consistent with the goals of social work practice and feminist ideology.

Frequently, there are obstacles in relationships that impede the achievement of the "five good things"; those "things" being a complex mix of elements that can easily be converted into negative consequences if we are involved in relationships that incur shame, violation, or trauma, resulting in a negative sense of self. The problem develops at the interface—the common contact barrier where interaction occurs. This meeting place symbolized each person's sense of being with the other, accompanied by the other's feelings and thoughts. What starts as a problem in the interaction often becomes internalized as a problem originating in the person and may be experienced as a personal failing. Women and girls in particular have been socialized to look to others for affirmation and value, placing them in a more vulnerable position to external criticism than boys and men (Surrey, 1987).

Self-esteem

An important question to ask oneself in making an assessment is: does this particular relationship give the client energy and power or does it deplete self-esteem and obstruct growth and development? Power and self-esteem are closely connected. People feel diminished when they are labeled in negative ways. However, when a person feels validated, accepted, respected, his or her sense of self flourishes, mobilizing inner resources for both problem solving and goal attainment. According to Jordan (1994), relational mutuality—mutual respect, mutual empathy, relatedness—can provide purpose and meaning in individuals' lives, while a lack of it can adversely affect self-esteem. Germain's (1991) definition of self-esteem fits well with the relational model and is still relevant today: "positive feeling about oneself acquired through experiences of relatedness, competence, and self-direction across the life course" (p. 26).

Traditional views suggest that our sense of competence and overall self-image is based on how we stack up against others. In other words, how we evaluate ourselves has to do with how we meet certain social and cultural ideals and standards set by our families, peers, mentors, community, and the larger society. The opinion others have of us is often internalized and incorporated into our self-esteem without our conscious awareness—particularly so with women (Walker, 2004). According to Judith Jordan (1991c), there may be more attentiveness to ideas and action for men, while women are often more focused on inner action, or a change of feelings which comes from "being with the other" (p. 4).

Anna's case: background and assessment

Competition is encouraged in bureaucracies like school systems and work places, where the hierarchical arrangement of power serves to get people to work harder. In this "separate self" model, an individual's sense of well-being can be derived from comparing one's self to others, and judging that self to be "better." These values of individual achievement and self-sufficiency are antithetical to the values of collaboration and connection rooted in the relational model. The following case illustrates how a competitive mother–daughter relationship and a competitive school environment can undermine the ability to develop a realistic and positive sense of self, contributing to feelings of low self-esteem and disempowerment.

Anna, a 20-year-old Caucasian college student from the West Coast, was enrolled in a dance conservatory program in the East Coast. She came to see me after her first episode of major clinical depression. Anna had lost 25 pounds, was listless, and had stopped attending classes. Her psychiatrist prescribed anti-depressant medication and advised her to take a six-month leave of absence from school. The college required that Anna receive weekly counseling as a condition of re-instatement.

During the first session, Anna seemed extremely self-conscious. She stated that she continuously judged herself in comparison to her classmates—she was either "much better" or "much worse." She strove for perfection, and felt that anything that fell short of that standard was unacceptable to her.

Anna's mother, Mrs. J., was also a dancer and choreographer who had given dance lessons in the home since Anna was young. Consequently, Anna had to compete for her mother's approval and attention with hundreds of other girls. She wanted to "stand out" and "be recognized" for her unique talents. Unfortunately, she never felt she succeeded. Anna's younger sister was also training to be a dancer. Her father, Mr. J., was a salesman and mostly concentrated on making a living for the family.

As she approached adolescence, Anna began to feel particularly vulnerable to rejection and ridicule. She stated that she felt different from others her age in her school and community because of her "artsy" way of dressing and her non-conformist behavior. Afraid she would be judged as "weird" by the other girls, she spent much of her time alone. The specialized performing arts college Anna attended was highly competitive, thereby intensifying the pressure she felt to succeed in the "real world" of dance. This atmosphere exacerbated Anna's anxiety and depression, leading her to further distance herself from her peers. She was in constant competition to prove to herself and, I suspect, to her mother, that she was worthwhile and a talented dancer. Even though her mother was miles away, Anna had internalized her critical voice.

Anna's case: analysis and discussion

The very continuity of mother–daughter ties allows for growth and maturation. However, there must be room for conflict and questioning, leading not to separation, but to self-differentiation (Kaplan et al., 1985). The mother-daughter relationship can be the basis for a positive mode of development. However, the child must be secure with herself and the relationship if she is to take a step toward changing the relationship in more complex and developmentally appropriate ways without disrupting underlying qualities of care and commitment. It seemed that Anna had had doubts about her career in dance that she could not openly acknowledge for fear of her mother's disappointment. It appeared that Mrs. J. had a difficult time accepting Anna unconditionally, and did not project the kind of confidence in her that Anna could incorporate into a positive self-image. Anna felt afraid that she would lose her mother's love and approval if her performance wasn't "perfect" or if she doubted her ability and desire to dance. Most of Anna's judgment of herself had been based on her mother's real or imagined approval or disapproval of her performance, and therefore the physical separation from home intensified Anna's doubts about her abilities.

Faculty members can be a source of personal validation for students; they can become an integral part of their human connection at school. Unfortunately, Anna felt that she did not get adequate feedback from the instructor whose work she most admired and respected. How could I help Anna build a more mutually supportive relational context with the other girls at her college, with her sister, and with her mother? How could she feel enough safety and care in her relationships so that she could risk bringing more of her own self and needs into authentic connection with others? How could I help her to be less harsh and more accepting of herself? These questions will be addressed in the next chapter on intervention.

The case of Lisa: a relational–cultural assessment

Cultural arrangements and power practices can divide people into groups of dominants and subordinates (Jordan et al., 2004). An analysis of cultural concepts may range from the use of power in a patriarchal society to issues of racial identity and growing up as a member of a minority group in which one's experiences are affected by gender, class, race, age, ethnicity, sexual orientation, and other markers that evoke oppression.

Assessing levels of felt marginalization and recognizing difference and diversity are intrinsic to a relational assessment. For example, groups and individuals that deviate from the dominant culture's ideals are devalued by the larger society. In turn, signs of withdrawal, lack of motivation to act on the environment, anger, and even despair may be manifested. This dynamic exerts a powerful influence on how people interact with others and may even create a vicious cycle of marginalization (Surrey, 1987). Clients from diverse cultural, economic, ethnic, racial, and other social groupings who have experienced prejudice may view the social worker (and the agency) with skepticism. This too should be factored into the assessment process.

The following case illustrates the lack of connection between a 15-year-old African-American adolescent and the primary social systems with which she interacted—family, school, and peers.

Lisa's mother, Mrs. M, called the counseling center requesting help for her 16-year-old daughter, whom she described as moody, explosive, and unhappy. Furthermore, Mrs. M was concerned about Lisa's grades, poor study habits, and lack of organizational skills. I initially met with Lisa and her mother together. Mrs. M is an attractive 48-year-old woman who appears both self-assured and somewhat anxious at the same time. Lisa is a moderately overweight, pleasant-looking teen who is quite engaging. She is bright and articulate, and displayed keen insight into herself and others.

Mrs. M expressed resentment about Lisa's lack of consideration of others at home, stating that "she leaves the house a mess and never picks up after herself." Mrs. M feels that her daughter makes excessive demands on her life, particularly in relation to her school work and social life. Mrs. M is a special-education teacher and is very invested in Lisa's success in school. However, she states that Lisa does her homework "at the last minute" and then wants help from her mother late at night. Mrs. M also stated that Lisa is intrusive when Mrs. M has friends over, leaving her little time for her own life. She wants Lisa to get involved in extracurricular activities at school, and to socialize with friends her own age. In essence, Mrs. M feels that Lisa is too dependent on her for her social and emotional needs.

Lisa feels that her mother does not listen to her, validate her feelings, or understand her needs and wants. Lisa admits that she has a hard time concentrating and thus procrastinates when it comes to doing her school work. She sees it as a problem and wants her mother to understand and empathize with her frustration rather than blame her for not doing well in school. Lisa is angry with both of her parents. Mr. M is a detective in the police force and is often at work or out of the house with his friends. When he is home he is emotionally unavailable and usually ignores Lisa. Lisa resents his lack of involvement in her life and verbalized that she would like to do more things with her father. Mrs. M also feels the lack of her husband's presence, since much of the burden of rearing Lisa falls on her shoulders.

Lisa agreed to see me individually on a weekly basis. In fact, she seemed quite eager to talk to someone. From time to time I saw Lisa with her mother and on a few occasions I saw Lisa with her father. Lisa fears that her parents, after being together for 16 years, will get divorced. Although she is aware that they share little physical affection or emotional intimacy, she enjoys the comfortable middle-class lifestyle, material possessions, and the sense of family they have been able to maintain. She says, "I don't want to be like my other friends who live in the housing development near my house and come from single parent families."

According to Lisa, her interest in academics and her middle-class lifestyle distance her from some of her peers who see her as "uncool" and "too white." Lisa is aware that she lives in a racist society where the majority culture has constructed stereotypes about black youth. Patricia Hill Collins refers to this idea as the concept of "controlling images" imposed by the dominant culture to define and marginalize subordinate groups (Jordan et al., 2004). These "images" often evoke race, gender, sexual orientation, or ethnicity. Lisa talks freely with me about the fact that she feels some of her teachers discriminate against the black kids and favor the white and Hispanic kids. She doesn't feel comfortable going to these teachers for extra help and, not surprisingly, she is doing poorly in these classes.

In middle school it was easier for Lisa to have relationships with youngsters from diverse backgrounds, but in high school it has become more difficult as the girls self-group based on social markers such as race, ethnicity, and sexual orientation. Furthermore, as Lisa moved into her middle teens her attempt to establish a personal identity was more intertwined with her racial identity, and there are few middle-income African-American students in her school with whom she can identify. In order to cope with her fear of rejection and social discomfort, she cuts herself off from school activities and heads home alone after school to "unwind."

During our subsequent sessions Lisa reiterated many of the same problems she stated in our beginning sessions—her distant relationship with her father, her strained relationship with her mother (whom she experiences as withholding and critical), and difficulty with her school work. She feels that her parents put great pressure on her to achieve at school and she does not want to share with them that she is having a particularly difficult time in her math and English classes.

A crisis erupted after I had been seeing Lisa for a couple of months. Mrs. M phoned in a very agitated state to tell me that Lisa had forged her signature on two English tests that she had failed. When I met with Lisa she too was clearly upset. She said, "I want to understand why I do what I do." She recognized that forging her mother's signature on her English tests was a way to avoid her parents' disapproval and was also perhaps a cry for help.

This incident seemed to open the way for Lisa to share thoughts and feelings she had previously kept to herself. She related that she felt unwanted and that she is responsible for her parents' troubled relationship. Although her mother denies this and claims that Lisa was premature and very much wanted, Lisa told me that she believes her parents only married because of her mother's pregnancy. This was and still is a family secret.

Analysis and discussion

Lisa lives in a lonely, confusing world in which she feels misunderstood. She experiences her parents as non-responsive to her needs and negates for her the legitimacy of her feelings and beliefs. Lisa's parents, by their own account, have an empty marriage, which contributes to a household that is devoid of hopeful connection. The difficulties Lisa's parents have with one another make her sad.

Every family has its share of secrets. However, secrecy can camouflage certain realities that contribute to patterns of systemic and chronic disconnections among family members (Miller & Stiver, 1997). Not only did the secrecy behind her mother's pregnancy cause Lisa to feel responsible for her parents' problems, but their distant relationship left her feeling alone, frightened, and confused. Her strategy for dealing with these feelings within the home was to alternate between being clingy, and being angry and explosive.

In this family, the lack of intimacy and mutuality between Mr. and Mrs. M affects all of the family members, and especially Lisa. Not having the opportunity to construct an open, reciprocal relationship with her parents exaggerates the normative power inequities that typically exist between adolescents and their parents. For example, while Lisa has a great need to be understood, her mother and father expend so much energy on trying to keep their relationship together for the sake of appearances, that it is difficult for them to be responsive to their daughter. Especially significant is the fact that Mrs. M is a wonderful role model in many ways, but Lisa doesn't believe she can win her mother's approval. In order to feel more powerful, Lisa is often angry and rude with her parents, teachers, and peers, causing them to withdraw from her. She is acutely aware of this interactional pattern and told me that although she doesn't want to change the essence of who she is, she would like to "soften her edges."

A supportive parent–child relationship is characterized by expressions of warmth and the absence of harsh criticism, and expressions of affection and good communication (Rutter, 1990). Interestingly, research findings show that major factors contributing to resilience in children and youth growing up in families characterized by marital discord have to do with the importance of relationships outside the family (Werner, 1989). Lisa has a loving and close relationship with her paternal grandparents who give freely of their time and money. This relationship compensates for the less than optimal one with her parents and supplies her with the protective factors predictive of her resilience. This mutually nurturing and caring relationship provides Lisa with a different relational image of herself and allows her to maximize her social potentials, her intelligence, caring, and warmth.

Social work best practices for assessment and planning

As a social worker you can enhance the assessment process through practicing the following techniques:

- Enable clients to become mutual partners in the assessment process. A dynamic collaboration process works best in achieving system goals.
- Assess levels of felt marginalization and recognize that difference and diversity are intrinsic to a relational assessment. Sensitivity to cultural diversity must be factored into a relational assessment; the ability to be self-reflective affects the worker's ability to gather data, analyze data, access the person-in-situation configuration, and derive goals and a plan of action.
- Use your assessment to evaluate the degree to which the client would benefit from the expression and fulfillment of dependency needs in life's relationships and under various circumstances, including the professional one. Assess the degree to which the client would benefit from striving toward more self-directed, autonomous functioning.

In summary, assessing clients' relationships in their total life space can help impact upon their self-esteem, sense of worth, and their ability to experience themselves as effective and empowered individuals within their environment.

6 Intervention
A relational–cultural point of view

The relational–cultural approach to clinical social work practice incorporates psychodynamic theories such as object relations, interpersonal, intersubjective, and self-psychology, and adds to the already existing literature on therapeutic relationship-building skills, cultural diversity, and practice interventions. The relational–cultural model embodies principles common to a relational and strengths-based perspective which fosters interpersonal relationship-building competencies and a greater sense of personal empowerment. The approach emphasizes the interactional nature of the intrapsychic, interpersonal, and macro social systems in which the client and clinician operate (Tosone, 2013).

According to William Borden, the relational paradigm rests on three core beliefs which are compatible with traditional practice wisdom and the values of social work practice: (1) the inherent capacity of a person to change; (2) the complexity and interdependence of human relationships and social life; and (3) the role of the professional relationship in the process of change (Borden, 2000). Since relational theory views all behavior as a result of the interaction between individuals and others in the social environment, interventions are directed at the intrapsychic, interpersonal, and social system levels.

Best relational practices include the following professional skills and values:

1   listening and responding;
2   focusing on the development of mutual empathy;
3   demonstrating responsiveness, authenticity, and the willingness to be impacted by the client;
4   moving toward mutuality in worker client relationship—the worker attempts to create a co-equal partnership, while minimizing power differences;
5   working with relational connections and disconnections in clients' lives;
6   working through and restructuring negative relational images;
7   fostering relational resilience; and
8   validating and incorporating clients' cultural and social context.

The case of Lisa: a relational–cultural context

In working with Lisa, who was introduced in Chapter 5, I utilized a variety of relational strategies to help her mobilize her inner strengths—her mature thought process, her accurate perception of her inner life and environment, and her desire and ability to engage in relationships. I also intervened in her family system to help them relate to one another in more mutually satisfying ways.

After several sessions I asked Lisa to write her thoughts, feelings, and experiences in a journal as a means of getting to know herself better and helping me to know her better. She regularly read me parts of her journal, which provided a wonderful vehicle for us to connect in a meaningful and non-threatening way. One day I asked Lisa to tell me about her friends, who were noticeably absent in her journal. This segued into a discussion about the kinds of "friends" she has. Although she hangs around with some kids in school, Lisa admits that they are more like acquaintances than a cohesive group of good friends in whom she can confide or trust. We spent some time talking about what creates a sense of closeness and trust with others, and what creates a sense of distance and mistrust in friendships. Some of the questions I posed to her were: How do you respond to your friends' needs? How do you show your friends you care and understand? How do your friends respond to your needs? How do they show you they care? Do you feel they understand you? Is your interest in each other reciprocal? Lisa and I discussed the importance of listening to others and having friends who are able to listen to her, willing to be there for her when she needs them, and vice versa.

Lisa was open to engaging in a therapeutic relationship with me and was willing to explore her major life issues. I helped her to think of new ways to express her feelings and thoughts to her parents when she felt they were not listening to her or understanding her. Reclaiming her voice in an appropriate manner helped increase her sense of empowerment and reduced her frustration. During one meeting with Lisa and her parents, they agreed to be referred to another social worker in my agency for couple's counseling. While they decided not to continue after a few sessions, Lisa came to understand that she did not "cause" whatever problems existed between her parents. This revelation helped to alleviate feelings of guilt which she had carried for a long time.

Lisa had stated on a few occasions that she wanted to spend more time with her father and readily accepted my suggestion to have a joint session with him. Mr. M agreed to meet with me and Lisa, during which time she was able to share her feelings of anger directly with him. Mr. M listened to Lisa and admitted that he often brings home feelings of frustration and anger from his stressful job as a detective, which helped Lisa not take her father's moods personally. They both expressed a desire to improve their relationship and made a date to go bowling the following week. Lisa was thrilled with this arrangement and let her father know she hoped they could do more things together in the future.

After meeting with Lisa and her dad, I met with Lisa and her mother. Both of them seemed to understand that they needed to listen to each other more carefully rather than to get defensive and "hotheaded" with each other. I talked with Mrs. M about the importance of being more empathic and accepting of Lisa. In her role as a special education teacher, mom was understanding and sensitive to the needs of her students. I appealed to these strengths, hoping to harness them in her relationship with her daughter. Lisa, on the other hand, needed to develop a greater sense of empathy for her mom in order to strengthen the bond and truly make it a mutual one. This will make it easier to establish a secure base with mom from which to differentiate herself and establish her own identity.

Through our relationship, Lisa came to appreciate the value of other relationships that she had in her life and worked harder to cultivate them. She reconnected with a cousin who lived a short distance away and a neighbor who was slightly older, but a compatible friend. I expressed to Lisa that I thought she was intelligent and insightful and that I really enjoyed working with her. Over time she became more motivated to do well in school and was excited about the possibility of going away to college in North Carolina where her maternal grandparents and cousins lived. With my support Lisa decided to take a math and an English course in summer school; and with the additional help of tutors her mother procured for her, she was pleased with the fact that she earned an A and a B in her summer courses.

Anna's case: intervention strategies

Anna, a college student studying at a dance conservatory about 3,000 miles from home, was introduced in the previous chapter on assessment. School was very stressful for Anna, as it was for Lisa, but in a different way. Anna was suffering from anxiety and had difficulty regulating her self-esteem. My overall plan was to help Anna feel more competent, help her regulate her self-esteem, enhance her sense of worth and self-direction, and help her to connect to others in her social network in more mutually satisfying ways. I worked with her to help her set her own performance standards, hoping to place more of the locus of control within herself. I empathized with the reality of the stress that she was experiencing, and validated the nature of the competitive world in which she was immersed, hoping this would increase her confidence and mitigate some of her self-criticism.

Validating the client's thoughts and feelings, and serving as a model of caring and concern, is especially crucial when working with a young woman who is at the juncture of late adolescence and young adulthood trying to carve out her own identity. As a way to help Anna gain a clearer sense of herself and to individuate, it was important to help her value her strengths, and to confront and accept the differences between herself, her mom, her sister, and the other co-eds in her program.

The turning point in the helping process came when Anna was chosen to be in the spring dance concert at her college and asked me if I would attend. Although I usually do not attend events outside of the agency with clients, after hearing how important it was to her, I decided to go. Also, since her family could not come as they lived 3,000 miles away, I thought it was particularly significant for Anna to have someone there just for her. At our session following the performance she asked me if I enjoyed the show. I shared my genuine pleasure in seeing her perform and told her how much I liked the production. Anna said that she was honestly surprised that I did not see the major mistake that she made at the beginning of her performance. At this point in our work together, I sensed some tension and felt there was a "disconnect" between us; I mentioned this to Anna, and asked her how she felt when I said that I did not notice her mistake. She stated that she did not feel that I was as observant or astute as someone who was trained in dance, and that therefore I would not have noticed her mistake. I shared with Anna that I felt she was minimizing my feedback, and that maybe this was more of an issue in terms of her own tendency to be hypercritical of herself.

Anna acknowledged that perhaps it was her own self-consciousness and unrealistic expectations that made her so unforgiving and hypercritical of herself; she expected either perfection or criticism—nothing in between. But after the interview I realized there was another issue, and that was that she was most disappointed that I was not her mother, the dance teacher. I was able to use this in the next session; I could empathize with her pain of not having her family present at her performance which touched her deeply.

Anna made an interesting comment toward the end of our next to last session before she was to return home for the summer. She said that although she knew she was smart, she always felt she lacked a social conscience. It was difficult for her to feel empathy for others or to relate to people with interest and care. As she developed more empathy for herself, she began to cultivate more empathy for others. Anna said, "You know I might even want to become a dance therapist so I can help others. I can't believe I can actually feel with others. I was never able to do that before." Through our mutual and authentic relationship, Anna slowly began to develop a greater self-acceptance of herself and a less critical self-introject. Now the challenge is for Anna to integrate a more realistic and positive self-concept as she moves into adulthood.

The importance of relational connections and contexts

Jean Baker Miller (1986) suggests that self-worth is a natural by-product of girls' and women's effectiveness in establishing, participating in, and maintaining mutually gratifying relationships. A shift in relational connections can be critical in realigning supports, creating a spiral of positive feelings, and an increased sense of strength in the agential self. In contrast to a sense of well-being, situations that contribute to low self-esteem are characterized by the sense of being unable to create movement or change.

The capacity to engage in a satisfying relationship with another person includes the sense of accomplishment that arises after completing a task successfully. Robert White (1963) theorized that humans possess an inborn drive toward mastery and competence. However, in order to achieve positive feelings about oneself the environment must provide the necessary conditions, opportunities, resources, and relationships. This proved to be true for Anna, the dance student.

The following is a list of ways in which practitioners may enhance the well-being and psycho-social functioning of clients while building self-esteem:

1 Explore the client's access to relationships that are responsive to his or her unique characteristics and temperament.
2 Help clients identify, establish, and expand relationships characterized by empowerment, empathy, genuineness, and responsiveness.
3 Encourage clients to identify and seek relationships that contribute to their learning opportunities and intellectual development (e.g. with mentors and teachers).
4 Assist clients to locate opportunities to enhance their sense of competence.
5 Explore clients' opportunities to create connections through peer groups, community groups, and self-help groups.
6 Examine the ways in which clients can make meaningful contributions to others through social action, mentoring, and community service.
7 Share feedback at moments of connection and disconnection between client and worker, and between client and external world.

Relational inventories

Fabio Folgheraiter (2007) frames relational social work as a style of work in professional practice, or a way of conceiving social helping in which the social worker facilitates and mobilizes social networks to help clients find ways to cope with difficulties experienced in living. For example, in the case of Jennifer, who was introduced in Chapter 5, the clinician connected with those in Jennifer's natural support network by selecting the key persons involved in solving the problem: her psychiatrist, lawyer, caseworker, brother, child psychologist, nursing colleagues, and the Administration for Children's Services (ACS) caseworker. They wrote letters and made conference calls, and the other nurses at work even accompanied her on visits with her son.

The quality and properties of one's social ties, social networks, community linkages, and personal relationships can allow for more effective problem solving and the ability to deal with societal inequities, feelings of powerlessness, and low self-esteem. A number of research studies are available that can help the worker evaluate the importance of relationships and social supports in women's lives.

The Relational Health Indices (RHI) (Liang et al., 1998) is one example of an exploratory study that is designed to assess growth fostering peer, mentor, and community relationships based on the relational–cultural theory set forth by feminist scholars at the Wellesley College Stone Center for Research on Women (see Appendix B of this book). The RHI was administered to a group of 450 first-year and senior students at a small women's liberal arts college. The research design included a set of three scales that assessed mentoring relationships, peer relationships, and community relationships separately. In particular, the concepts of self-disclosure and openness, authenticity, empowerment/zest, and the ability to deal with difference or conflict, were found to be associated with growth-fostering relationships.

The quality of one's connection to community, peers, and mentors was predictive of depression and loneliness scores. Self-esteem was associated with all three relational types. These outcomes suggest that the clinician needs to pay close attention to those relationships that: (1) are mutual and respectful, (2) can facilitate emotional resiliency and coping strategies, and (3) provide motivation for reaching out for additional social supports.

I adapted the following questions from the Relational Scale Questionnaire (RSQ) developed by Griffin and Bartholomew (1994) in my work with many of my clients and often use them as a semi-structured open-ended questionnaire to help focus the interview and gather information that may shed light on the nature and quantity of mutual satisfying relationships:

1 Are there people in your life on whom you feel you can depend?
2 Are there people in your life who you feel can depend on you?
3 How important is it for you to feel independent?
4 How comfortable are you depending on other people?
5 How easy is it for you to get emotionally close to another person?
6 How comfortable are you with being alone?
7 Do you think you get as much as you give in your close relationships?
8 Do you think your relationships are characterized
9 Do you think that others value you as much as you value them?
10 Do you feel you are able to express your feelings, thoughts, and opinions clearly?

11 Do you feel you are listened to?
12 Do you feel you listen to the other person's point of view?
13 Are others energized by their relationship with you?
14 Do you feel supported and encouraged in your close relationships?
15 Do you feel you are able to give support and encouragement to others?
16 Do you feel you can be genuine and real in your close relationships?
17 Do you feel others are honest and real with you?
18 Do you feel you are able to negotiate difference and conflict in your relationships?
19 Do you feel you are open to accepting and dealing with conflict and differences in your relationships?

In my work with Anna, her responses to these questions were enlightening not only for me, but for Anna as well. In addition to other co-eds, faculty mentors can be a source of personal validation for students; they can become an integral part of their human connection at school. Unfortunately, Anna was not able to find a mentor who could provide useful feedback and support. However, she was able to see more clearly that her lack of connectedness with others in the campus community left her without a sense of belonging, which in turn contributed to her loneliness and depression. Her characteristic style of relating was to use distancing maneuvers related to her anxiety about how she would be judged by others. The therapist encouraged Anna to reach out to faculty members as a way to get to know them better and to get feedback. Gaining new insights about herself, she grew more motivated to become an integral part of her campus community.

Think of an individual with whom you work. Imagine you are that person. How do you think he or she would answer the above questions from the RSQ? What additional information might you gather from his or her responses that could guide your intervention techniques?

A support group for women with eating disordered behaviors

Through the coordinated efforts of parents, interested individuals, and political leaders, an eating disorder support group was formed and funded in a mental health clinic in a small city in the Northeast. The group that emerged from these efforts consisted of 8 women aged 24 to 55, each of whom had a DSM-4 diagnosis of anorexia, bulimia, or eating disorder NOS. In addition to a history of restricting food intake and/or engaging in bingeing and purging behaviors, all individuals had at least one other psychiatric diagnosis such as generalized anxiety disorder, bipolar disorder, depression, borderline personality disorder, post-traumatic stress disorder, or other psychiatric disorders. Most reported their own earlier abuse of alcohol or other substances though none had concurrent alcohol or other substance dependence issues while in the group; and all but one had attended 12 step programs in the past. A trauma history that included physical and/or sexual abuse was evident in the backgrounds of at least six of the members; these women also reported they were raised by a parent or caregiver who had been alcohol dependent and had a probable or diagnosed mental illness.

A significant number of group members had poor to moderate ability with daily functioning; while two were employed, most were unemployed or on disability. Members of the group reported low self-esteem, and difficulty naming feelings and regulating uncomfortable affective states which resulted in their diminished capacity to soothe themselves, and all members indicated they felt isolated from others.

The group met for 10-week sessions that each lasted for two hours, and it continued to meet throughout the year with several breaks for holiday periods. New members were generally allowed into the group up until the third session. It was required of each person to have her own therapist throughout the time she participated in the group.

At the start of each 10-week session, members were given a phone and email list (anyone could opt out of putting her personal information on the list), and encouraged by the facilitator to communicate with each other by phone or email during times of distress or at other times when feedback from group members was sought. Communication between members outside of group sessions afforded each individual an opportunity to create a friendship network. Among other things, this support network involved the exchange of feelings and thoughts, the coordinating of schedules and the planning of trips to a local coffee shop or other activity (e.g. a communal hike) that occurred several times over the course of a year.

Relational theory as the facilitator's theoretical base

The group leader's theoretical orientation included the incorporation of concepts and the use of models from dialectical behavior therapy (Linehan, 1993), stages of change theory (Prochaska et al., 2006) and motivational interviewing (W.R. Miller & Rollnick, 2002). However her primary theoretical framework was relational–cultural therapy (RCT) which posits that movement toward mutuality, empowerment, and connection is seen as the basis of healthy human development. From the vantage point of the group members who reported feeling trapped by years of difficulty with eating issues, relational therapy offers a way out of the condemned isolation and the feelings of powerlessness they report by helping them recognize and move toward relationships that foster their own and other's growth.

Strategies of disconnection

According to the work of relational theorists and practitioners Jean Baker Miller and Irene Stiver (1997), symptoms associated with eating disorders (such as the restricting of food and liquid, cutting, laxative abuse, and other self-harming behaviors) can be considered strategies of disconnection. These strategies are used by eating disordered group members to disconnect from their own needs and feelings while attempting to maintain some sort of relationship with family members, spouses, partners or others. Women who relate to self and significant others by using strategies of disconnection increase their isolation and dependence upon disordered eating behaviors, on the one hand. On the other hand, they are attempting to create a means by which to preserve a view of themselves as being in relation to important people in their lives, while in actuality they are alienated and cut off from others. This usually happens when interactions with significant others lack mutual empathy, are fraught with disappointment, and sometimes even danger or violation (Tantillo et al., 2001). Indeed, the facilitator's acceptance of these strategies of disconnection and her invitation to examine and gradually change them was a major part of the ongoing work of the group.

Relational images

In response to these losses of connection, Miller and Stiver (1997) theorized that women formed "relational images" constructed from early interactions with others. As women develop images of themselves, they also create a set of beliefs about why relationships are the way they are. These images can often determine a person's sense of herself or himself, and embody what each person expects to happen in future relationships as well. In other words, people act in ways that confirm their early internalized relational self-image. They also noted that women are capable of experiencing a combination of conflicting relational images which can compound their confusion as they approach or avoid interactions with others. What is most concerning is that negative relational images can become the source of a lack of relational competence and worth and support strategies of disconnection people employ throughout their life—disordered eating being one of them.

The RCT group facilitator brings with her an awareness of the role of the central relational paradox (yearning for connection yet keeping oneself out of connection so that relationships are maintained). She also helps group members unpack the meaning of the relational images that have influenced how they interpret their own needs, feelings, and interactions with others, and guides their burgeoning understanding of how these strategies further perpetuate the disordered eating, low self-esteem, and profound sense of isolation members report at the outset of the group. Through an emphasis on relational experience within and outside the group, the facilitator models and maintains an accepting attitude toward herself and group members that fosters a mutually empathic and mutually empowering, growth-fostering environment.

When used in the context of a group for members with disordered eating, this relational concept suggests that participants:

- keep large parts of themselves out of connection with others which results in their inability to reap the benefits of connection;
- restrict the formation of new ways of experiencing themselves; and
- rely on old patterns of interaction which allow for relationships to be maintained at the cost of their own personal growth and development.

Case vignette 1: group illustration of relational images

At the fourth group meeting Yvonne entered the room carrying a heavy backpack which she swung on the table before her. She began emptying its contents of eight books, several notepads, and a pen. Yvonne carefully arranged the books around her with the backpack in the middle and, opening her notebook, sat ready with pen in hand. The group leader, Sue, noted that Yvonne had done this at each of the previous three sessions and hoped the members might bring this up in the group. That evening Sue observed that Maggie, another group member, was covering her mouth with her hands, while watching Yvonne intensely. When the group commenced, Sue asked Maggie if she had something to share with Yvonne. Maggie gazed at the leader, said nothing, and lowered her eyes. Sue reminded Maggie and the other group members that recovery and healing were more likely when group members shared honestly how they were affected by other members' thoughts, feelings, and behavior.

Knowing how difficult it would be for Maggie to "unsilence" herself, which she had been doing for years to avoid conflict with others, Sue brought up a relational image Maggie had earlier stated in the group of making herself "invisible" so as not to show neediness or draw attention to herself. Sue, the group leader, pointed out that she was doing this now. Maggie said, "I learned to take care of myself as a kid. When my mother was drunk or locked in her room when I came home from school, I went into the woods behind our house to be safe." After a few minutes of silence, Maggie asked for help from the group. Other members mentioned times when they felt speaking up could be dangerous and could result in disconnections from their siblings and/or parents. Sue encouraged the members to speak openly about past relational experiences and they parlayed that into experiences with group members. Yvonne was both expectant and apprehensive when she asked the group for feedback. With the support and encouragement of the group and leader, Maggie looked at Yvonne and said, "You've built a fortress of books around yourself ... it's like you're refusing to let anyone in." Yvonne seemed saddened by this comment saying she needed the books there to bolster her identity; their presence at the table made her feel she was smart. She related that years of academic difficulties left her feeling she was "stupid." It was eventually discovered through testing that her learning disability and attention deficit disorder had never been properly diagnosed. "Now that I take medicine I can understand what I read, and I am trying to make up for lost time by reading a lot of books."

Sue pointed out to Yvonne that although she might think the books protect her from the shame she has felt in her life, they also create a boundary which intensifies her loneliness and further makes her feel disconnected from other people. Several members empathized with Yvonne's feeling of humiliation and shame, and spoke of relational disconnections they had experienced as children. Another group member said she empathized with Yvonne's feelings and understood her experiences in school because she too had struggled with similar academic problems and repeatedly fought self-doubts about herself. She praised Yvonne for her courage and determination to seek help for her learning disorder and attention deficit diagnosis.

Prompted by Yvonne's sharing her feelings of sadness and shame in response to Maggie's "fortress of books" comment, the facilitator invited further exchange among members of their own use of relational images and strategies of disconnection. The honest yet painful discussion that followed resulted in what appeared to have a paradoxical outcome: nearing the end of the group session, two members mentioned their own feelings of heightened vulnerability, which they attributed to a spike of negative feelings toward themselves. The members reported they were more able to see their disordered eating behavior as a way of "still being stuck" in old patterns which they believed protected themselves against the experience of serious and chronic disconnection in significant relationships with family, friends, and life partners. Yet despite these painful feelings that group discussion brought up, the facilitator noticed most members left the room talking quietly to each other, while several others offered and received hugs.

Using a relational–cultural framework, the group facilitator:

- explained how a child's walling herself off from potentially injurious relationships was really a self-protection solution to feelings of shame, inadequacy, and powerlessness;

- showed how these protective solutions often became strategies of disconnection that allowed the child a means to maintain familial and other relationships while distancing the child from her own needs and feelings;
- discussed how self-empathy was one of the foundational elements of healthy relationships; something they would continue to discuss in group;
- helped Maggie and other members to recognize how courageous she had been by communicating her observations with group members; and
- helped foster a sense of mutual empathy, connection, and willingness by others to share painful experiences with lesser fear of the group's judgment or rejection.

Reflecting on this session the following week at a staff meeting, Sue noted that the groundwork had been laid for a new sense of mutual purpose and aid nurtured by the feelings of mutual empathy that the women began to experience for each other.

Case vignette 2: group illustration of disconnection

As was her practice, Sue began session eight with a relaxation exercise. Asking the group to focus mindfully on their breathing with their eyes closed, she began reading from a script and guided them through a 10-minute exercise. When the exercise ended, she asked the group for feedback on their experiences. Marley responded stridently saying "I was totally turned off by it. The minute you used the phrase about us being 'large women' I told myself that I was done with this. I turned off to you and got nothing from this at all." Within seconds a chorus of others repeated similar reactions, including one comment by a group member who added that she believed Sue had been insensitive to their body image worries.

Sue openly engaged all members of the group and encouraged them to continue to share all of their reactions to the exercise. After they spoke, Sue admitted she felt badly about not picking up on the phrase and altering the reading before presenting it to the group. She explained that she had interpreted the phrase to mean women's large capacity to share and nurture themselves and others. She thanked them for bringing it to her attention, and apologized for appearing insensitive to the feelings of the group participants. However, she asked the group members to expand on what they were thinking and feeling once they heard her use the phrase. Lorna, like Marley, had a negative reaction, and said that she found herself questioning Sue's judgment; she was uncomfortable holding on to these negative thoughts and began to doubt her own reaction. Sandra expressed feelings of guilt saying she hadn't wanted to be annoyed with Sue and wondered if she had been wrong to verbalize her response to the exercise. She and Reesa both agreed that they were afraid Sue would stop liking them since they agreed with Marley, and wondered about returning to the group.

Sue decided to use the disconnection that had just occurred between herself and group members as an opportunity to remind the women that relationships are fraught with potential for disconnections and reconnections. She continued that people have different perspectives, and it is important to look for opportunities to repair the disconnections that keep eating disorders in place. Open and honest dialogue can present a relational opportunity to repair and rebuild relationships that facilitate recovery. Sue assured them that she was not angry; in fact, she appreciated their feedback, and thanked them for their honest sharing. At that point, she became aware that the energy in the room had changed and the group agreed. Giving them the opportunity to name feelings and share thoughts encouraged mutual empathy among group members and validated their respective responses.

The RCT group facilitator helped create growth-fostering relationships within the group and between herself and group members by:

- encouraging group members to verbalize a relational image that captured their vision of themselves and their relationship with others; and the meaning they attached to this image;
- asking group members to consider earlier experiences in their lives when they felt a disconnection from themselves and others;
- inviting group members to share the strategies they used for dealing with the disconnection (e.g. silencing, restricting food intake, overeating, cutting, etc.);
- demonstrating that repair is possible through mutual sharing of thoughts and feelings; and
- accepting the members' feedback and responding in an authentic manner.

After reflecting on the "large women" session, Sue told her clinical supervisor that she now saw it as having been a turning point in the life of the group. The conflict members had over verbalizing their displeasure with her was overcome; they were able to genuinely share their thoughts and feelings, which increased empathy among all members, created a greater sense of solidarity among them, and increased the level of trust they had toward the leader. From that session on, which Sue referred to as "the night of the gradual awakening," members became more willing to share painful relational images and strategies they employed to stay tethered to unhealthy relationships.

In summary, the relational clinician can enhance the intervention process by practicing the following techniques:

- Systematically explore and reach for clients' feelings about those significant relationships in which there has been a disconnection. Keep in mind that those relationships which are absent from a person's life may be more clinically relevant than those which are present.
- Establish linkages to social networks in the community to reduce isolation and maximize the opportunities for healthy, growth-producing connections.
- Direct actions toward assessing the nature and quality of social supports so that institutional resources, community programs, and organization that support and enhance the client's coping and adaptive capacities can be mobilized.

7 Ethics and values
A feminist perspective

Every practice paradigm in social work is supported by a constellation of values and a code of ethics that is reflected in the mission, theoretical and empirical base, practice skills and techniques, and general philosophy and outlook of that paradigm. These ethics and values are not merely abstract concepts—they hold everyday importance for all social workers. A brief overview of the values and ethics that guide the feminist relational approach to practice incorporates many of the core principles presented in this book.

Professional values and ethics, which share important principles with philosophical systems of feminism, have an impact on almost everything we do, what we ask, how we intervene, and how we interpret what we find. Values and ethics are the underpinnings of the social work profession and play an important role in how social workers respond to situations, make decisions, and enact their roles on a day-to-day basis (Phillips & Straussner, 2002). The National Association of Social Workers (NASW) Code of Ethics is "based on the fundamental values of the social work profession that include the worth, dignity, and uniqueness of all persons as well as their rights and opportunities" (1999, p. 1). Three core values identified in the code of ethics and expressed in the feminist relational model are:

1   the inherent worth and dignity of the human being;
2   mutual respect, acceptance, and caring; and
3   self-determination.

The inherent worth and dignity of the human being

Feminist values of interdependence and interconnectedness, relational commitment, and a sense of morality that encompasses mutual compassion and care correspond to the traditional social work value that each individual has inherent dignity, sharing common needs with others (Collins, 1986). Since its inception, social work has had to justify its value base to other male-dominated professions that regard caring as "unscientific" and merely an extension of the female role (Freedberg, 1993). There are few fixed rules in the practice of social work. Ethical systems must take into account culture, context, personality, the nature of the client–worker relationship, and the nature of the client's connections to others.

Most central to the feminist relational perspective is the notion discussed in Chapter 3 of mutuality, a unifying concept that underlies both the practice and ethics of social work. Genero and her colleagues (1992) refer to mutuality as the "bi-directional movement of feelings, thoughts, and activity between persons in relationships" (p. 36). This suggests an openness to the constant changing patterns of worker and client responding to and affecting each other's state, with a special awareness of the other's subjective experience (Jordan, 1986). Simply stated, when one is the recipient of concern, attention, and care, one is in a better position to give these back, thereby enhancing the quality of all of one's relationships.

Empathy combined with mutuality allows the worker to develop a sense of how the client thinks and feels, so that working together, worker and client can co-create a shared relational experience. Surrey (1997) states that "Mutuality describes a creative process, in which openness to change allows something new to happen, building on the different contributions of each person" (p. 42). Encouraging a sense of mutuality maximizes feelings of competence, which leads to an increased sense of worth and dignity. In sum, mutuality entails mutual appreciation, communication, sharing, and the commitment of each being there for the other. With the ongoing experience of relationships characterized by mutuality and relational bonding, real care and concern emerge. The motivation to connect with others, rather than to merely be gratified by others, represents a basic shift from traditional approaches (Miller & Stiver, 1997).

We do not live in a world that always respects mutuality. Whenever one group has power over another, disconnections and violations may result. The mutuality model, in contrast to the power-over model, aims to enhance the individual's self-respect and supports the worth and dignity of each human being by helping them to become aware of the power imbalances that exist and the ways in which they can address them. However, even in relationships where there is an unequal distribution of power such as teacher–student, parent–child, inmate–guard, listening to the other's experience, learning about the other's perspective, asking questions, sharing thoughts and feelings, or telling stories can help equalize the playing field.

Mutuality offers each person in the relational system an opportunity to contribute actively on different levels, minimizing power differentials and enhancing respect and self-esteem. For example, when social workers acknowledge mistakes they make and their uncertainties, showing they are "human" may increase trust between the worker and client.

Mutual respect, acceptance, and caring

Mutuality involves being engaged in a growing connection with another person. Mutual respect grows out of healthy connections. As the relationship unfolds, honoring the uniqueness of each other becomes integral to the growth of mutual respect. Reflection can be used to identify, explore, and affirm a client's strengths, abilities, and uniqueness. The social work practitioner acts as an empathic investigator, helping the client get to know him or herself better, and engaging him or her in a relationship in which each enjoys being part of the experience, being moved, being understood, and being accepted by the other, and feeling with the other. When the worker is open to his or her own feelings, he or she can more easily resonate with the client, increasing the mutual impact they can have on each other.

Social work is about care. In fact caring about others is considered the very foundation of social work (Rhodes, 1985). Psychologist and philosopher Willard Gaylin (1978, p. 33) defines caring as:

The protective, parental, tender aspects of loving found among peers, child to parent, friend to friend, lover to lover, person to animal. The parent–child aspect of caring is an essential paradigm whose presence is necessary for the diffusion of this human quality into the other relational aspects of life.

It is difficult to define *care* in absolute terms; it is related to an act of well doing, a moral obligation, or the responsibility to be there for another. Sometimes caring is a motive that drives behavior. But it always involves an emotional component, a responsiveness *to*, an investment in, and a concern for another (Noddings, 1984). Although it differs from culture to culture, care almost always involves providing for the social, economic, physical, and/or emotional needs of someone else (Kolb, 2003). It is an act of doing that can extend beyond an emotional response.

Self-determination

Part of the social worker's repertoire of skills and techniques may involve helping clients to clarify an ethical code of values that will help guide their actions. Decision-making processes often depend on the ability of the social worker to mobilize the client's wants and needs and decision-making abilities. The great philosopher Immanuel Kant asserted that it is a person's right to determine his or her destiny (Loewenberg & Dolgoff, 1992). Maximizing opportunities for clients to make decisions about their own lives is inherent in applying this principle to social work practice (Freedberg, 1989). However, self-determination is not an absolute right. Much of the time this concept, when applied to practice, is trumped by the lack of alternatives in a modern, hierarchical society, one in which certain people are limited by opportunity and privilege, laws and norms.

According to the National Association of Social Workers' Code of Ethics (1999), "Social workers respect and promote the right of clients to self-determination and assist clients in their effort to identify and clarify their goals" (p. 4). In many ways, the notion of self-determination has become a source of one of the most common and perplexing dilemmas for social workers in working with women (Abramson, 1985). Women's available choices have historically been limited as a result of their diminished social status, their sense of autonomy compromised because of the oppression rooted in the social structures of a patriarchal society. Sometimes, without realizing it, females internalize the expectation that they should suppress their own needs in order to accommodate to the needs of others. One of the primary tasks for the social worker is to help the client get in touch with her own will so she can have a better chance to actualize herself.

Before women, or any oppressed group for that matter, can be helped to determine their life course they must be empowered to believe they have the right to choose. The seeds of self-empowerment may be planted in the client–worker relationship, which then may be transferred onto other relationships in the client's life. To accomplish this objective, the feminist relational school emphasizes the practitioner's role in fostering mutuality and maximizing client participation in the change process. Mobilizing client motivation and determination lies at the heart of the strengths perspective, as well as the feminist relational approach to practice.

Patricia Hill Collins (1990) notes that the feminist method of understanding and explaining experience rests on the concept that "the personal is political." Similarly, the feminist relational approach offers a way of analyzing life and politics and the interaction between them. A political analysis of personal experience fits well with both the feminist relational approach and the ecological-systems perspective, which entails understanding how the individual and the social environment intersect. As women and other marginalized groups come to know themselves better, and understand the role played by the political hierarchy in defining their reality, they may ultimately change their conception of the goals they set out to achieve for themselves in life. For social workers, helping these groups achieve a more conscious recognition of the different influences that guide their behaviors may ultimately lead them to discover their own voices and enhance self-determination.

The case of Theresa

The following case vignette demonstrates how cultural values can influence the relational process and create a practice dilemma for the clinician whose personal background is different from that of the client. The clinician walks a fine line in her commitment to respecting the client's values, accepting her choices, and helping her to make the best decision for herself while minimizing hurt for others.

Theresa is a Latina woman in her mid-fifties and the worker is a white female and in her early sixties. Although Theresa was acculturated to the American way of life, she held onto many of the traditional values and customs of her Hispanic heritage, particularly her Catholicism, attending church on a regular basis; religion, or a sense of spirituality, informs the traditional Hispanic experience (Gonzalez, n.d.). Theresa was very close to her family—her mother, father, sister, and niece, as well as her two sons. Having recently gone through a divorce, her connection *to* them and the support she received *from* them were more important than ever. According to Dr. Manny Gonzalez, loyalty to the nuclear and extended family, or *familism*, often supersedes the focus on individual needs. Giving respect (*respeto*) to others, especially to those in authority, as well as maintaining respect for traditional social roles, are key to the individual's sense of identity (Garcia-Preto, 2005). The clinician must be mindful and respectful of relational meanings in the client's life, not only in terms of self-identity, but also in terms of cultural identity, both of which plays a large part in determining an individual's self-perception.

Theresa had been seeing the therapist overall for three years—but in two one-and-a-half-year intervals. The first time she abruptly terminated by not showing and not returning the worker's phone call. About a year later she returned, with the presenting problem being that she had separated from her husband of twenty-five years and was contemplating divorce. The clinician and client had developed a solid working relationship over the years, both having an appreciation for each other's culture. The therapist provided support for Theresa's impending divorce, facilitated her adaptation to a new job as a business education instructor in a community college, and helped her deal with the "empty nest" syndrome after one son left for college and the other recently got married; an easy rapport soon developed again.

After several sessions Theresa disclosed to the worker that she had been having a sexual relationship with her friend Diane for the past year. Theresa had talked about Diane many times in the past, and they seemed to have a close relationship, one which provided Theresa with a good deal of support and companionship. However, after Theresa met a man, Ralph, she broke off her relationship with Diane, stating that she did not see herself cultivating and living a lesbian lifestyle for the rest of her life. Theresa had known Ralph for about twenty years through her previous job, and although she had not seen him for a while, he had recently contacted her. She said Ralph made her laugh, she was happy being with him, and she enjoyed sex with him.

Theresa felt a great deal of shame about her involvement with Diane, vowing to never share this with her parents or children as it went against her religious values and her family's belief system. She was clear that she wanted to maintain a friendship with Diane, but nothing more, preferring instead to see if she could build a life together with Ralph. Sharing this "secret" with the therapist afforded her some relief, despite her fear of disapproval.

Perhaps most important to the treatment was the fact that the worker had to understand the cultural and ethical issues that prompted Theresa's decision to cut off her relationship with Diane. The clinician had been involved in the women's movement and other liberal causes, and strongly supported the notion of "choice." Although the clinician was ready to help Theresa by supporting her relationship with Diane and coming out to her family, this was not what the client wanted. After further exploration, it was clear that Theresa was committed to living her romantic and sexual life more in keeping with traditional cultural values, ones in which she felt "no need to hide anymore." The clinician, mindful of the client's desires, understood her decision and the values that shaped it, and supported her.

In the past year, the client had experienced a "disconnect" from her mother and father lasting for about a year. Both Theresa and her mother were strong-willed, and if they were able to talk things out with each other, the loss of connection could have been avoided. With help from the clinician, Theresa was able to repair this relationship, which resulted in a stronger connection than they had previously. The centrality of her relationship with her mother and father (i.e. the love and protection she received from her parents) was more important to her than challenging the status quo. In this case, the therapist had to respect the client's decision and all the factors those are based on even though they may have conflicted with the clinician's own belief system. Hiersteiner and Peterson (1999) state, "Although care-centered practice focuses social workers' attention on clients, it maintains both clients' presenting problem and society's responses" (p. 243). *Confianza*, or the intimacy and familiarity in a relationship, supports the bond of trust that must be established and maintained if a therapeutic relationship is to be a positive one (Gonzalez, n.d.).

What became obvious to the clinician was Theresa's pattern in handling conflict in relationships—she abruptly terminated her relationship with this therapist after one year of working together; she terminated her relationship with her parents after a dispute about their desire to live close to her and her family; and now she was ending her sexual relationship with Diane so precipitously. Theresa has a difficult time asserting herself, especially with people she cares about; she becomes overcome with guilt, and rather than possibly hurt them or cause them disappointment, she just "walks away."

Relevant to this case is what I call the "ethics of fairness," that is the responsibility one has for another person. The clinician felt that if Theresa was going to end her romantic relationship with Diane, it should be done in a direct way, making it clear that Theresa wanted to maintain the friendship but end the sexual relationship. This was something Diane had a very difficult time accepting. Rather than confront her own guilt, and afraid to hurt Diane, Theresa chose to withdraw instead of engaging in conflict. According to Miller & Surrey (1997), authentic relationships offer us the gift of conflict—the opportunity for the emergence of something new. A premise of RCT is that the therapist works to facilitate mutual responsibility, not only in the client–worker relationship, but those relationships that offer the potential for empowerment, or a sense of effectiveness (Bergman & Surrey, 2004). Our work eventually resulted in Theresa resuming her connection to Diane, albeit in a different, but mutually constructive way.

In reality, most client–worker situations present dilemmas that raise the following questions:

1   How do we maintain our responsibility for the therapeutic relationship and our responsibility to protect the client; and yet move away from a hierarchical or paternalistic stance in the relationship if necessary?
2   When our own emotional response takes us out of connection with the client and when acknowledging that response could be experienced as intrusive to the client, how do we decide what to do?
3   From an ethical perspective, when is it "safe enough" to take some risks, Safe for whom? And when is too much safety potentially harmful for the client as well as to the quality of the therapeutic relationship?
4   How do we maintain our responsibility for the therapeutic relationship yet make honest statements to the client without causing him or her to withdraw from the relationship?

A feminist ethic of care

The term "feminist ethic of care" can be used interchangeably with the term "care ethic" because both prioritize concern for relationship and both recognize that there are innate dilemmas in the concept of care. A feminist or relational ethic of care, based on a care-based perspective, contributes to the value, theory, and practice base of social work. Care ethics:

•   begins with the assumption of human connectedness;
•   stresses the role of empathy and the role of emotions as part of the caring connection; and
•   emphasizes the importance of building community.

(Noddings, 2012)

Noddings believes that care ethics speak to the importance of reciprocity and mutuality in the roles of both carer and cared-for in establishing and maintaining that relationship. Irene Stiver (1997) highlights the multiple meanings in the act of caring, observing that the giving of care sometimes involves arrangements characterized by dependency, and at other times there is a certain degree of interdependency. However, all participants in a relationship are impacted by the act of caring. Problems may arise, such as in a caretaking situation, when one person has a much greater need for care than the other. The imbalance that is created in the relationship may lead to frustration, anger, and depression. For example, when one person suffers from severe illness or a handicap, and the cared-for is unable to respond in a way that completes the relation, the work of the carer becomes more and more difficult. Carers in this position need the support of a caring community to sustain them (Noddings 1984).

Boszormenyi-Nagy (1987) theorized that when accountability is not attended to, and when the give and take of relationships become imbalanced, the result may impact on physical or mental health problems including stagnant and/or destructive relationships, and psychosomatic illness. For example, in formal settings such as the workplace, when people feel entitled to something they are not getting, this deep feeling of "unfairness" may leave them blind to the distress of others, and can lead to anger and even rage. Research has shown how using the power of the peer group in the implementation of an ethic of care in a drug-free therapeutic community can counteract tendencies to resist help and change. The stability of community life depended on a communal value system that encouraged honesty, commitment to the welfare of others, mutual respect and fairness, and a belief in the human potential to change. Residents of the drug-free community were required to show responsible concern: they assumed responsibility for the recovery of peers. Everyone had to "buy into" this relational value system to overcome their substance abuse problem. This vision embraces the idea that affirming others in their struggle to recover is also caring about them (Soyez et al., 2004). In essence, what is definitive about care seems to be a perspective of taking the other's needs as the starting point of what must be done.

The social context that frames any relationship must be taken into account to understand the exchange of care that takes place. Contextual theory is a theory which argues that the context in which human activity takes place—the time, the space, and the place in the sequence of events—is crucial to the nature of that activity (Gangamma et al., 2012). Inherent in contextual theory is the notion of relational ethics, which is concerned with the overarching balance of give and take within relationships. The emphasis on the balance of fairness in relationships through consideration of relational ethics distinguishes this approach from other integrative approaches which looks at healing individual pain in the context of social systems, in this case, the family system (Boszormenyi-Nagy, 1987). When relational ethics are balanced, and each person can focus on giving and receiving respect, concern, care, and sometimes even love and nurture, instilling a commitment to care can further enhance the quality of the relationship and develop a greater sense of self and integrity in the individuals involved.

In the therapeutic relationship, the expression of caring on the part of the clinician has sometimes been viewed as interfering with the neutrality required in the healing process. This "interference" has also been labeled as countertransference, a term which implies that the worker is projecting his or her own needs and feelings from earlier relationships onto the client. However, if the clinician is too cautious, the authentic connection that ultimately can prove so powerful can be hindered. In essence, the client needs to feel cared about. Caring is not only therapeutic, but also serves as a critical dimension of one's ability to adapt to complex environments, to establish and sustain relationships, and to enhance one's base of support. All of these abilities may support a stronger sense of self and more effective coping strategies.

A feminist ethic of care emphasizes a longing for connection as the motivational force that underpins the development of women who have been socialized into a set of caregiving roles. Women are more inclined to define themselves in relation to others; the desire to "do good," to assume responsibility for others, and to execute appropriate judgment is embedded in their conception of care and morality (Noddings,

1984). Some women hold a vision of relationships that gives rise to an ethic of justice and care—that everyone will be treated equally and will be entitled to a basic sense of belonging and love. What gives this vision a feminist cast is its emphasis on the investment of feeling in the other person. According to Noddings, this ethic is rooted in relatedness, receptivity, and responsibility for the other.

Reciprocity and mutuality are important in relational ethics. Martin Buber wrote, "One should not try to dilute the meaning of the relation: relation is reciprocity" (1970, p. 58). But the reciprocity that care ethicists refer to is not the contractual reciprocity in traditional ethics ("you scratch my back and I'll scratch yours"). Simply put, it is the mutual recognition and appreciation of response. The response often provides further information about his or her needs and interests, and how the carer might deepen or broaden the relation. The response provides the building blocks for the construction of a continuing caring relation (Noddings, 2012). As with parents of newborns, it usually is not until the infant can respond back with some sort of recognition that the parent and child have bonded in a truly meaningful way in which each recognizes the other as part of him or herself. This kind of natural caring increases a sense of loyalty and strengthens the relationship.

Noddings argues that the carer must exhibit engrossment and motivational displacement, and the person who is cared for must respond in some way to the caring (1984). She terms this idea of mutuality as engrossment, referring to thinking about someone in order to gain a greater understanding of him or her. Engrossment is necessary for caring because an individual's personal and physical situation must be understood before the one caring can determine the appropriateness of any action. Engrossment does not suggest a deep fixation on the others; it requires attention needed to understand the position of the other. In relational caring, we are mainly interested in the caring relation, not so much in the merit of the carer. When things go wrong, the cared-for does not recognize the effort of the carer, as is often the case in the social worker-client relationship, and the carer (social worker) must have the maturity to understand this and try something else.

Many times, women who assume the caretaker role do so because they believe that they are following a normative role prescription. Conforming to the feminist ethic of care, the "morally mature" person understands and can negotiate the balance between caring for the self and caring for others (Freedberg, 1993). When a female client experiences conflict between competing responsibilities, the social worker may need to help her accept the idea that caring for herself is not selfish— that she may continue to care for others while continuing to care for herself at the same time.

Like Noddings, Carol Gilligan provided a conceptual framework through which to analyze an ethic of care. The central thesis of Gilligan's landmark book *In a Different Voice* (1982) is that a longing for connection is an important motivational force that underlies the moral development of women and results in the desire to care for others. Individuals have been socialized in a society that has largely bifurcated male and female expectations in relation to the commitment to care. Girls and women have been taught to define their sense of self and self-worth in relation to their nurturing and caretaking roles; boys and men have been taught to define their sense of self-worth in relation to their roles as providers and protectors.

Gilligan (1982) found that females moved in and out of three moral frames of reference over their life space:

- Level I: overemphasis on an interest in themselves.
- Level II: overemphasis on an interest in others.
- Level III: a balance between a healthy interest in themselves and a healthy interest in others.

It is important for social workers to provide opportunities for all clients to experience a sense of connection, continuity, and belonging that will allow them to create a socially responsible image of themselves.

A second development in the scholarship on the ethics of care is represented in the work of Joan Tronto (1993). For Tronto, an ethic of care cannot be understood unless it is placed in a moral and political context. Her definition of care is as follows:

> On the most general level, we suggest that caring be viewed as a species activity that includes everything we do to maintain, continue, and repair our world so that we can live in it as best as possible.
>
> (Tronto, 1993, p. 103)

Moreover, she sees the activity of caring as largely defined culturally and it will vary from group to group. What is definitive about care seems to be a perspective of taking the other's needs as the starting point of what must be done (Featherstone & Morris, 2012). Compassionate, care-centered practice focuses attention on maintaining a careful balance on the individual client and on salient social, political, and environmental factors that influence both clients' problems and society's responses, all with a sense of moral responsibility to the community at large (Hiersteiner & Peterson, 1999). This position is consistent with the legacy of social work and the leaders who shaped our profession. In the 1930s and 1940s, Bertha Capen Reynolds and other social workers in the rank-and-file movement committed themselves to the union movement, not only to better wages and working conditions, but as an important vehicle to connect workers to each other and to the services they used.

However, today the principle of caring and compassion in social work too often lacks the context of a community of shared values. A model of mutuality and interdependence is a vision that the profession must continue to strive for, not only as a philosophy, but in order to invigorate our rich legacy of caring and responsibility for others; one that is vitally important, now more than ever.

Appendix A

The Mutual Psychological Development Questionnaire (MPDQ) Project Report, Stone Center, Wellesley College, Wellesley, MA

Nancy Genero, Jean Baker Miller, and Janet Surrey

We would like you to tell us about your relationship with your spouse or partner. By partner we mean a person with whom you live or with whom you have a steady relationship.

<u>If married</u>, how many years?

What is your spouse's age?

<u>If not married</u>, how long have you known your partner?

What is your partner's age?

Are you currently living with your partner? (Please circle)   YES   NO

In this section we would like to explore certain aspects of your relationship with your spouse or partner. Using the scale below, please tell us your best estimate of how often you and your spouse/partner experience each of the following:

1 = Never	3 = Occasionally	5 = Most of the time
2 = Rarely	4 = More often than not	6 = All the time

When we talk about things that matter to my spouse/partner, I am likely to ...

Be receptive	1	2	3	4	5	6
Get impatient	1	2	3	4	5	6
Try to understand	1	2	3	4	5	6
Get bored	1	2	3	4	5	6
Feel moved	1	2	3	4	5	6
Avoid being honest	1	2	3	4	5	6
Be open-minded	1	2	3	4	5	6
Get discouraged	1	2	3	4	5	6
Get involved	1	2	3	4	5	6
Have difficulty listening	1	2	3	4	5	6
Feel energized by our conversation	1	2	3	4	5	6

When we talk about things that matter to me, my spouse/partner is likely to …

Pick up on my feelings	1	2	3	4	5	6
Feel like we're not getting anywhere	1	2	3	4	5	6
Show an interest	1	2	3	4	5	6
Get frustrated	1	2	3	4	5	6
Share similar experiences	1	2	3	4	5	6
Keep feelings inside	1	2	3	4	5	6
Respect my point of view	1	2	3	4	5	6
Change the subject	1	2	3	4	5	6
See the humor in things	1	2	3	4	5	6
Feel down	1	2	3	4	5	6
Express an opinion clearly	1	2	3	4	5	6

This questionnaire was reproduced with permission from Nancy Genero.

Appendix B
The Relational Health Indices:
An exploratory study

Belle Liang, Catherine Taylor, Linda M. Williams,
Allison Tracy, Judith Jordan, and Jean Baker Miller

FINAL SELECTION OF ITEMS FOR RELATIONAL HEALTH INDICES

(0 = never; 1 = seldom; 2 = sometimes; 3 = often; 4 = always)

PEER ZEST/EMPOWERMENT

16 I feel positively changed by my friend.
18 After a conversation with my friend, I feel uplifted.
19 I feel as though I know myself better through my connection with my friend.

AUTHENTICITY

29 Even when I have difficult things to share, I can be honest and real with my friend.
31 I am truthful with my friend even when it might hurt his/her feelings.
32 I can tell my friend when he/she has hurt my feelings.

DIFFERENCES

14 I accept the differences between my friend and myself.
15 Even when we argue, I try to understand how he/she feels about the subject.

EMPATHY/ENGAGEMENT

10 It is important to us to make our friendship grow.
23 The more time I spend with my friend, the closer I feel to him/her.
25 My friendship inspires me to seek other friendships like this one.

COMMUNITY ZEST/EMPOWERMENT

4   Being a member of this community gives me a better sense of who I am.
5   I feel better about myself after my interactions with this community.

6   I feel mobilized to personal action after meetings within this community.

AUTHENTICITY

13 It doesn't feel comfortable to be genuinely myself in this community.
24 Members of this community are not free to be themselves.
25 There are parts of myself I feel I must hide from this community.

DIFFERENCES

20 Differences of opinion among members are accepted within this community.
21 Members of this community can express different opinions without feeling judged and rejected.
27 Differences of background among members are not accepted within this community.

EMPATHY/ENGAGEMENT

7   I feel understood by members of this community.
8   If members of this community know something is bothering me, they ask me about it.
9   It seems as if people in this community really like me as a person.

MENTOR ZEST/EMPOWERMENT

12 I feel uplifted and energized by conversations with my mentor.
13 My mentor helps me to feel I can do things I didn't think I could do.
14 I feel as though I know myself better because of my mentor.

AUTHENTICITY

21 I can genuinely be myself with my mentor.
22 I believe my mentor values me as a whole person (e.g. professionally/academically and personally).
23 My mentor gives me constructive and honest feedback.

DIFFERENCES

28 My mentor makes me feel responsible for meeting his/her needs.
29 My mentor places excessive demands on me.

EMPATHY/ENGAGEMENT

18   My mentor shares personal experiences, feelings and thoughts with me.
19   It is important to me to foster the growth of this relationship.
34   My mentor shares stories about his/her own experience with me in a way that enhances my life.

Reproduced with permission from Belle Liang.

References

Abramson, M. (1985). The autonomy–paternalism dilemma in social work practice. *Social Casework, 66*(7), 387–393.

Addams, J. (1960). *A centennial reader.* New York: Macmillan.

Agnew, E.N. (2004). *From charity to social reform.* Urbana, IL: University of Chicago Press.

Astin, H.S. (1967). Assessment of empathic ability by means of a situational test. *Journal of Counseling Psychology, 14*(1), 57–60.

Banks, A.E. (2010). Developing the capacity to connect. *Work in Progress*, No. 107. Wellesley, MA: Center for Research on Women Working Paper Series.

Barnhart, C. (Ed.). (1966). *American college dictionary.* 2nd Edition. New York: Random House.

Basch, M.F. (1988). *Understanding psychotherapy.* New York: Basic Books.

Beck, B. (1977). The community center as a human service organization. In *Encyclopedia of settlements and community centers*, 11, 1262–1266.

Beebe, B. & Lachmann, F.M. (2002). *Infant research and adult treatment.* Hillsdale, NJ: The Analytic Press.

Belenky, M.F., Clinchy, B.M., Goldberger, N.R., & Tarule, J.M. (1986). *Women's ways of knowing.* New York: Basic Books.

Bellak, L. & Goldsmith, L.A. (1984). *The broad scope of ego function assessment.* New York: Wiley.

Benjamin, J. (1988). *Bonds of love.* New York: Pantheon.

Benjamin, J. (1998). *Shadow of the other: Intersubjectivity and gender in psychoanalysis.* New York: Routledge.

Berger, D.M. (1987). *Clinical empathy.* Northvale, NJ: Jason Aronson.

Bergman, S. (1991). Men's psychological development: A relational perspective. *Work In Progress*, No. 39. Wellesley, MA: Stone Center Working Paper Series.

Bergman, S.J. & Surrey, J.L. (2004). Couples therapy: A relational approach. In J.V. Jordan, M. Walker, & L.M. Hartling (Eds.), *The complexity of connection* (pp. 167–194). New York: Guilford Press.

Berzoff, J. (1989). From separation to connection: Shifts in understanding women's development. *Affilia: Journal of Women and Social Work, 4*(1), 45–58.

Berzoff, J., Flanagan, L.M., & Hertz, P. (2011). *Inside out and outside in: Psychodynamic clinical theory and practice in contemporary multicultural contexts.* 3rd Edition. Lanham, MD: Rowan & Littlefield.

Biestek, F.P. (1957). *The casework relationship.* Chicago: Loyola University Press.

Bohart, A.C. & Greenberg, L.S. (Eds.). (1997). *Empathy reconsidered: New directions in psychotherapy.* Washington, DC: American Psychological Association.

Borden, W. (2000). The relational paradigm in contemporary psychoanalysis: Toward a psychodynamically informed social work perspective. *Social Service Review* (September), 364–379.

Boszormenyi-Nagy, I. (1987). *Foundations of contextual therapy*. New York: Routledge.

Bowlby, J. (1969). *Attachment and loss, Vol I*. New York: Basic Books.

Boyle, S.W., Hull, G.H., Mather, J. H., Smith, L.L., & Farley, W.O. (2006). *Direct practice in social work*. Boston: Allyn & Bacon.

Brazelton, T.B., Koslowski, B., & Main, M. (1974). *The origins of reciprocity: The early mother–infant interaction*. Hoboken, NJ: Wiley & Sons.

Brenner, C. (1974). *An elementary textbook of psychoanalysis*. New York: Doubleday.

Buber, M. (1970). *I and thou*. New York: Scribner & Son.

Casius, C. (Ed.). (1950). *A comparison of diagnostic and functional casework concepts*. New York: Family Service Association of America.

Chodorow, N. (1978). *The reproduction of mothering*. Berkeley, CA: University of California Press.

Chodorow, N.J. (1994). *Femininity, masculinities, sexualities*. Lexington, KY: University Press.

Collins, B.G. (1986). Defining feminist social work. *Social Work, 31*(3), 214–221.

Collins, P.H. (1990). *Black feminist thought: Knowledge, consciousness, and the politics of empowerment*. New York: Routledge.

Compton, B.R., Galaway, B., & Cournoyer, B.R. (2005). *Social work processes*. 7th Edition. Belmont, CA: Brooks/Cole.

Cooper, M. & Lesser, J.G. (2005). *Clinical social work: An integrated approach*. 2nd Edition. Boston: Allyn & Bacon.

Cozolino, T. (2006). *The neuroscience of human relationships: Attachment and the developing brain*. New York: Norton.

Dewane, C.J. (2006). Use of self: A primer revisited. *Clinical Social Work Journal, 34*(4), 543–558.

Dinnerstein, D. (1997) *The Mermaid and the Minotaur*. New York: Harper Books.

Dyche, L. & Zayas, L.H. (2001). Cross-cultural empathy and training the contemporary psychotherapist. *Clinical Social Work Journal, 29*(3), 245–258.

Ehrenreich, J. (1985). *The altruist imagination*. Ithaca, NY: Cornell University Press.

Eisenberg, N. & Strayer, J. (1987). Critical issues in the study of empathy. In N. Eisenberg & J. Strayer (Eds.), *Empathy and development* (pp. 3–16). Cambridge, UK: Cambridge University Press.

Elwert, F. & Christakis, N.S. (2008). The effects of widowhood on mortality by the causes of death of both spouses. *American Journal of Public Health, 98*(11), 2092–2098.

Erikson, E.H. (1950). *Childhood and society*. New York: Norton.

Erikson, E.H. (1968). *Identity: Youth and crisis*. London: Faber & Faber.

Farley, O.W., Smith, L.L., & Boyle, S.W. (2008). *Introduction to social work*. 11th Edition. Boston: Allyn and Bacon.

Featherstone, B. & Morris, K. (2012). Feminist ethics of care. In M. Gray, J. Midgley, & S. Webb (Eds.), *The Sage handbook of social work* (pp. 341–355). Thousand Oaks, CA: Sage Publications.

Finlayson, A.D. (1937). The diagnostic process in continuing treatment. *Social Casework, 18*, 228–233.

Folgheraiter, F. (2007). Relational social work: Principles and practices. *Social Policy and Society, 6*(2), 265–274.

Fonagy, P. (2001). *Attachment theory and psychoanalysis*. New York: Other Press.

Fox, R., (2001). *Elements of the helping process*. Binghamton, NY: The Haworth Press.

Freedberg, S. (1984). *Bertha Capen Reynolds: A woman out of step with her times*. Unpublished doctoral dissertation, Columbia University.

Freedberg, S. (1989). Self-determination: Historical perspectives and effects on current practice. *Social Work, 34*(1), 33–38.

Freedberg, S. (1993). The feminine ethic of care and the professionalization of social work. *Social Work, 38*(5), 535–540.

Frey, L. (2013) Relational–cultural therapy: Theory, research, and application to counseling competencies, *Professional Psychology: Research and Practice*, 44(3), 177–185.

Gangamma, R., Bartle-Haring, S., & Glebova, T. (2012). A study of contextual therapy theory's relational ethics in couples therapy. *Family Relations*, 61, 825–835.

Garcia-Preto, N. (2005). Latino families: An overview. In M. McGoldrick, J. Giordano, N. Garcia-Preto (Eds.), *Ethnicity and family therapy* (pp. 153–166). 3rd Edition. New York: Guilford Press.

Garrett, A. (1958). The worker-client relationship. In H.J. Parad (Ed.). *Ego psychology and dynamic casework* (p. 53). New York: Family Service Association of America.

Gaylin, W. (1978). The limits of benevolence. In W. Gaylin, I.M. Glaser, & D. Rothman (Eds.), *Doing good* (pp. 1–39). New York: Pantheon.

Genero, N.P., Miller, J.B., Surrey, J. (1992). The mutual psychological development questionnaire. *Work in Progress*, No.1. Wellesley, MA: Stone Center Working Paper Series.

Germain, C.B. (1970). Casework and science: A scientific encounter. In R.W. Roberts & R.H. Nee (Eds.), *Theories of social casework* (pp. 3–33). Chicago: University of Chicago Press.

Germain, C.B. (1991). *Human behavior in the social environment: An ecological view*. New York: Columbia University Press.

Germain, C. & Gitterman, A. (1986). The life model to social work practice approach revisited. In F.J. Turner (Ed.), *Social work treatment interlocking approaches* (pp. 618–645). 3rd Edition. New York: The Free Press.

Germain, C.B. & Gitterman, A. (1996). *The life model of social work practice*. 2nd Edition. New York: Columbia University Press.

Gilligan, C. (1982). *In a different voice: Psychological theory and women's development*. Cambridge, MA: Harvard University Press.

Goldstein, E. (1984). *Ego psychology and social work practice*. New York: The Free Press.

Goldstein, E.G. (1996). In F. Turner (Ed.), *Social work treatment* (pp. 168–191). 4th Edition. New York: Free Press.

Goldstein, E.G. (2001). *Object relations theory and self psychology in social work practice*. New York: The Free Press.

Goldstein, E. G., Miehls, D., & Ringel, S. (2009). *Advanced clinical social work practice*. New York: Columbia University Press.

Gonzalez, M. (n.d.). Clinical practice with Hispanic patients: A relational–cultural approach. Unpublished manuscript, Silberman School of Social Work, Hunter College, City University of New York, New York, NY.

Greenberg, J.R. & Mitchell, S.A. (1983). *Object relations in psychoanalytic theory*. Cambridge, MA: Harvard University Press.

Griffin, D.W. & Bartholomew, K. (1994). The metaphysics of measurement: The case of adult attachment. In K. Bartholomew & D. Perlman (Eds.), *Advances in personal relationships Vol. 5: Attachment processes in adulthood* (pp. 17–52). London: Jessica Kingsley Publishers.

Guntrip, H.J.S. (1971). *Psychoanalytic theory, therapy, and the self*. New York: Basic Books.

Hall-Flavin, D.K. (2012) (expert opinion). Mayo Clinic, Rochester, MN. August 27, 2012.

Herman, J. (1997). *Trauma and recovery*. New York: Basic Books.

Hamilton, G. (1951). *Theory and practice of social casework*. New York: Columbia University Press.

Hepworth, D.H., Rooney, R.H., Rooney, G.D., Strom-Gottfried, K., & Larsen, J. (2006). *Direct social work practice, theory, and skills*. Belmont, CA: Thomson.

Herman. J. (1997). *Trauma and recovery*. New York: Basic Books.

Hiersteiner, C. & Peterson, K.J. (1999). Crafting a usable past: The care-centered practice narrative in social work. *Affilia, 14*(2), 144–161.

Hill, O. (1875). *Homes of the London poor*. New York: Macmillan.

Hoffman, M. (1997). Sex differences in empathy and related behaviors. *Psychological Bulletin, 84*(4), 712–722.

Hollis, F. (1964). *Casework: A psychosocial therapy*. 1st Edition. New York: Random House.

Hollis, F. (1981). *Casework: A psychosocial therapy*. 3rd Edition. New York: Random House.

Howell, E. (1981). Psychological reactions of postpartum women. In E. Howell & M. Bayes (Eds.), *Women's mental health* (pp. 340–347). New York: Basic Books.

Jordan, J.V. (1983). Empathy in the mother-daughter relationship. In J.V. Jordan, J.L. Surrey, & A. Kaplan (Eds.), *Women and empathy* (pp. 2–5). Wellesley, MA: The Stone Center.

Jordan, J.V. (1984). *Empathy and self-boundaries*. Wellesley, MA: Wellesley Centers for Women.

Jordan, J.V. (1985). Self in relation: A theory of women's development. *Work in Progress*, No. 13. Wellesley, MA: Stone Center Working Paper Series.

Jordan, J.V. (1986). The meaning of mutuality. *Work in Progress*, No. 23. Wellesley, MA: Stone Center Working Paper Series.

Jordan, J.V. (1989). *Relational development: Therapeutic implications of empathy and shame*. Wellesley, MA: The Stone Center.

Jordan, J.V. (1991a). Empathy and self boundaries. In J.V. Jordan, A.G. Kaplan, J.B. Miller, I.P. Stiver, & J.L. Surrey (Eds.), *Women's growth in connection* (pp. 67–80). New York: The Guilford Press.

Jordan, J.V. (1991b). Empathy, mutuality and therapeutic change: Clinical implications of a relational model. In J.V. Jordan, A.G. Kaplan, J.B. Miller, I.P. Stiver, & J.L. Surrey (Eds.), *Women's growth in connection* (pp. 283–290). New York: The Guilford Press.

Jordan, J.V. (1991c). The meaning of mutuality. In J.V. Jordan, A.G. Kaplan, J.B. Miller, I.P. Stiver, & J.L. Surrey (Eds.), *Women's growth in connection* (pp. 8–96). New York: The Guilford Press.

Jordan, J.V. (1991d). *The movement of mutuality and power*. Wellesley, MA: Wellesley Centers for Women.

Jordan, J.V. (1994). *A relational perspective on self-esteem*. Wellesley, MA: Wellesley Centers for Women.

Jordan, J.V. (1997a). A relational perspective for understanding women's development. In J.V. Jordan (Ed.), *Women's growth in diversity: More writings from the Stone Center* (pp. 9–24). New York: The Guilford Press.

Jordan, J.V. (1997b). Clarity in connection: Empathic knowing, desire, and sexuality. In J.V. Jordan (Ed.), *Women's growth in diversity: More writings from the Stone Center* (pp. 50–73). New York: The Guilford Press.

Jordan, J.V. (1997c). Relational development: Therapeutic implications of empathy and shame. In J.V. Jordan (Ed.), *Women's growth in diversity: More writings from the Stone Center* (pp. 138–161). New York: The Guilford Press.

Jordan, J.V. (1997d). The relational model as a source of empowerment for women. In M.R. Walsh (Ed.), *Women, men, and gender: Ongoing debates* (pp. 373–382). New Haven, CT: Yale University Press.

Jordan, J.V. (2004). Toward competence and connection. In J.V. Jordan, M. Walker, & L.M. Hartling (Eds.), *The complexity of connection: Writings from the Stone Center's Jean Baker Miller training institute* (pp. 11–28). New York: The Guilford Press.

Jordan, J.V. & Dooley, C. (2000). *Relational practice in action: A group manual*. Wellesley, MA: Wellesley Centers for Women.

Jordan, J.V. & Hartling, L.M. (2002). New developments in relational cultural theory. *Work in Progress*, No. 29. Wellesley, MA: Stone Center Working Paper Series.

Jordan, J.V., Kaplan, A.G., Miller, J.B., Stiver, I.P., & Surrey, J.L. (1991a). *Women's growth in connection: Writings from the Stone Center*. New York: The Guilford Press.

Jordan, J.V., Surrey, J.L., & Kaplan, A.G. (1991b). Women and empathy: Implications for psychological development and psychotherapy. In J.V. Jordan, A.G. Kaplan, J.B. Miller, I.P. Stiver, & J.L. Surrey (Eds.), *Women's growth in connection* (pp. 27–50). New York: The Guilford Press.

Jordan, J.V., Walker, M., & Hartling, L.M. (Eds.). (2004). *The complexity of connection: Writings from the Stone Center's Jean Baker Miller training institute.* New York: The Guildord Press.

Kaplan, A.G. (1988). *Dichotomous thought and relational processes in therapy.* Wellesley, MA: Wellesley Centers for Women.

Kaplan, A.G. (1991a). Female or male therapists for women: New formulations. In J.V. Jordan, A.G. Kaplan, J.B. Miller, I.P. Stiver, & J.L. Surrey (Eds.), *Women's growth in connection* (pp. 268–282). New York: The Guilford Press.

Kaplan, A.G. (1991b). The "self-in-relation": Implications for depression in women. In J.V. Jordan, A.G. Kaplan, J.B. Miller, I.P. Stiver, & J.L. Surrey (Eds.), *Women's growth in connection* (pp. 206–222). New York: The Guilford Press.

Kaplan, A.G., Klein, R., & Gleason, N. (1985). Women's self development in late adolescence. *Work in Progress*, No. 17. Wellesley, MA: Stone Center Working Paper Series.

Kaplan, A.G., Klein, R., & Gleason, N. (1991). Women's self development in late adolescence. In J.V. Jordan, A.G. Kaplan, J.B. Miller, I.P. Stiver, & J.L. Surrey (Eds.), *Women's growth in connection* (pp. 122–142). New York: The Guilford Press.

Keefe, T. (1976). The development of empathic skill: A study. *Journal of Education for Social Work, 15*(2), 30–38.

Kernberg, O.F. (1976). *Object relations theory and clinical psychoanalysis.* Northvale, NJ: Jason Aronson.

Kimmel, M. (Ed.). (2004). *The gendered society.* New York: Oxford University Press.

Kohlberg, L. (1981). *Essays on moral development, Vol I: The philosophy of moral development.* New York: Harper & Row.

Kohut, H. (1977). *The restoration of the self.* New York: International Universities Press.

Kolb, P. (2003). *Caring for our elders.* New York: Columbia University Press.

Kuhn, T.S. (1970). *The structure of scientific revolutions.* Chicago: University of Chicago Press.

Lacan, J. (1985). *Feminine sexuality.* New York: W.W. Norton & Company.

Levine, E.R. (2002). Glossary. In A.R. Roberts & G.J. Greene (Eds.), *Social work desk reference* (pp. 829–849). New York: Oxford University Press.

Levinson, D.J. (1978). *The seasons of a man's life.* New York: Ballentine Books.

Liang, B., Taylor, C., Williams, L.M., Tracy, A., Jordan, J.V., & Miller, J.B. (1998). *The relational health Indices: An exploratory study.* Wellesley, MA: Wellesley Centers for Women.

Linehan, M. (1993). *Cognitive-behavioral treatment of borderline personality disorder.* New York: Guilford Press.

Loewenberg, F.M. & Dolgoff, R. (1992). *Ethical decisions for social work practice.* Itasca, IL: F.E. Peacock Publishers.

Lubove, R. (1969). *Professional altruist: The emergence of social work as a career 1880–1930.* New York: Atheneum.

Mahler, M.S., Pine, F., & Bergman, A. (1975). *The psychological birth of the human infant: Symbiosis and individuation.* New York: Basic Books.

Marsh, J.C. (2005). Social work: Help starts here. *Social Work, 50*(3), 195–196.

Meyer, C.H. (1993). *Assessment in social work practice.* New York: Columbia University Press.

Miller, J.B. (1976). *Toward a new psychology of women.* Boston: Beacon Press.

Miller, J.B. (1986). *What do we mean by relationships?* Wellesley, MA: The Stone Center.

Miller, J.B. (1991a). The construction of anger in women and men. In J.V. Jordan, A.G. Kaplan, J.B. Miller, I.P. Stiver, & J.L. Surrey (Eds.), *Women's growth in connection* (pp. 181–196). New York: The Guilford Press.

Miller, J.B. (1991b). The development of women's sense of self. In J.V. Jordan, A.G. Kaplan, J.B. Miller, I.P. Stiver, & J.L. Surrey (Eds.), *Women's growth in connection* (pp. 11–26). New York: The Guilford Press.

Miller, J.B. (1991c). Women and power. In J.V. Jordan, A.G. Kaplan, J.B. Miller, I.P. Stiver, & J.L. Surrey (Eds.), *Women's growth in connection* (pp. 197–205). New York: The Guilford Press.

Miller, J.B. & Stiver, I.P. (1991). *A relational reframing of therapy*. Wellesley, MA: The Stone Center.

Miller, J.B. & Stiver, I.P. (1995). *Relational images and their meaning in psychotherapy*. Wellesley, MA: The Stone Center.

Miller, J.B. & Stiver, I.P. (1997). *The healing connection: How women form relationships in therapy and in life*. Boston: Beacon Press.

Miller, J.B. & Surrey, J.L. (1997). Revisioning women's anger: The personal and the global. In J.V. Jordan (Ed.), *Women's growth in diversity: More writings from the Stone Center* (pp. 199–216). New York: The Guilford Press.

Miller, J.B., Jordan, J.V., Stiver, I.P., Walker, M., Surrey, J.L., & Eldridge, N.S. (1999). *Therapists' authenticity*. Wellesley, MA: The Stone Center.

Miller, W.R. & Rollnick, S. (2002). *Motivational interviewing preparing people to change addictive behaviors*. New York: The Guilford Press.

Minahan, A. (Ed.). (1986). *Encyclopedia of social work*. 18th Edition. Washington, DC: National Association of Social Workers.

Mitchell, S.A. (1988). *Relational concepts in psychoanalysis: An integration*. Cambridge, MA: Harvard University Press.

Mitchell, S.A. & Black, M.J. (1995). *Freud and beyond: A history of modern psychoanalytic thought*. New York: Basic Books.

National Association of Social Workers (NASW). (1999). *Code of ethics*. Washington, DC: NASW.

Noddings, N. (1984). *Caring: A feminine approach to ethics and moral education*. Berkeley, CA: University of California Press.

Noddings, N. (2012). The language of care ethics. *Knowledge Quest, 40*(5), 52–56.

Perlman, H.H. (1957). *Casework: A problem-solving process*. Chicago: University of Chicago Press.

Perlman, H.H. (1979). *Relationship: The heart of helping people*. Chicago: University of Chicago Press.

Phillips, N.K. & Straussner, L.A.S. (2002). *Urban social work*. Boston: Allyn & Bacon.

Pinderhughes, E. (1979). Teaching empathy in cross-cultural social work. *Social Work, 24*(4), 312–316.

Prochaska, J.O., Norcross, J.C., & DiClemente, C.C. (2006). *Changing for good a revolutionary six stage program for overcoming bad habits and moving your life positively*. New York: Harper Collins.

Pumphrey, R. E. & Pumphrey, M. W. (1961). *The heritage of American social work*. New York: Columbia University Press.

Raines, J.C. (1990). Empathy in clinical social work. *Clinical Social Work Journal, 18*(1), 57–72.

Raines, J.C. (1996). Self-disclosure in clinical social work. *Clinical Social Work Journal, 24*(4), 357–375.

Reynolds, B.C. (1934). *Between client and community: a study in responsibility in social case work*. New York: Oriole Editions.

Reynolds, B.C. (1951). *Social work and social living*. Silver Spring, MD: National Association of Social Workers.

Rhodes, M.L. (1985). Gilligan's theory of moral development as applied to social work. *Social Work, 30*(2), 101–106.

Richmond, M.E. (1899). *Friendly visiting among the poor: A handbook for charity workers*. New York: Charity Organization Society of New York.

Richmond, M.E. (1917). *Social diagnosis*. New York: Russell Sage.

Richmond, M.E. (1922). *What is social casework? An introductory description.* New York: Russell Sage Foundation.

Robinson, V.P. (1930). *A changing psychology in social casework.* Chapel Hill, NC: University of North Carolina Press.

Rogers, C. (1951). *Client centered therapy.* New York: Houghton Mifflin.

Rowe, C.E. & Mac Isaac, D.S. (1991). *Empathic attunement: The technique of psychoanalytic self psychology.* Northvale, NJ: Jason Aronson.

Rutter, M. (1990). Psychosocial resilience and protective mechanisms. In J. Rolf, A.S. Masten, D. Cicchetti, K.H. Nuechterlein, & S. Weintraub (Eds.), *Risk and protective factors in the development of psychopathology,* (pp. 181–214). New York: Cambridge University Press.

Shulman, L. (2006) *The skills of helping individuals, families, groups, and communities.* Belmont, CA: Thomson.

Siegel, D.J. (2012). *Interpersonal neurobiology.* New York: W.W. Norton.

Silverstein, R., Buxbaum, L.B., Tuttle, A., Knudson-Martin, C. & Huenergardt, D. (2006). What does it mean to be relational? A framework for assessment and practice. *Family Process, 45*(4), 391–405.

Smalley, R. (1970). The functional approach to casework. In R. W. Roberts and R.H. Nee (Eds.), *Theories of social casework* (pp. 77–129). Chicago: University of Chicago Press.

Smith, K.F., Goodman, L., & Glenn, C. (2006). The full-frame approach: A new response to marginalized women left behind by specialized services. *American Journal of Orthospychiatry, 76*(4), 489–502.

Solomon, A. (2012). *Far from the tree.* New York: Scribner.

Soyez, V., Tatrai, H., Broekaert, E. & Bracke, R. (2004). The implementation of contextual therapy in the therapeutic community: A case study. *Journal of Family Therapy, 26*(3), 286–305.

Specht, H. (1994). *Unfaithful angels.* New York: Free Press.

Spencer, R. (2000). *A comparison of relational psychologies.* Wellesley, MA: Wellesley Centers for Women.

St. Clair, M. & Wigren, J. (2004). *Object relations and self psychology: An introduction.* Belmont, CA: Thomson/Brooks/Cole.

Stern, D.N. (1985). *The interpersonal world of the infant: A view from psychoanalysis and development psychology.* New York: Basic Books.

Stiver, I.P. (1991a). Beyond the Oedipus complex: Mothers and daughters. In J.V. Jordan, A.G. Kaplan, J.B. Miller, I.P. Stiver, & J.L. Surrey (Eds.), *Women's growth in connection* (pp. 97 –121). New York: The Guilford Press.

Stiver, I.P. (1991b). The meaning of care: Reframing treatment models. In J.V. Jordan, A.G. Kaplan, J.B. Miller, I.P. Stiver, & J.L. Surrey (Eds.), *Women's growth in connection* (pp. 250–267). New York: The Guilford Press.

Stiver, I.P. (1991c). The meanings of "dependency" in female–male relationships. In J.V. Jordan, A.G. Kaplan, J.B. Miller, I.P. Stiver, & J.L. Surrey (Eds.), *Women's growth in connection* (pp. 143–161). New York: The Guilford Press.

Stiver, I.P. (1997). A relational approach to therapeutic impasses. In J.V. Jordan (Ed.), *Women's growth in diversity: More writings from the Stone Center* (pp. 288–310). New York: The Guilford Press.

Stiver, I.P. & Miller, J.B. (1988). *From depression to sadness in women's psychotherapy.* Wellesely, MA: The Stone Center.

Stolorow, R.D., Atwood, G.E., & Brandchaft, B. (Eds.). (1994). *The intersubjective perspective.* Northvale, NJ: Jason Aronson.

Sullivan, H.S. (1940). *Conceptions of modern psychology.* New York: William Allison White Psychiatric Foundation.

Surrey, J.L. (1987). *Relationships and empowerment.* Wellesley, MA: The Stone Center.

Surrey, J.L. (1991a). Eating patterns as a reflection of women's development. In J.V. Jordan, A.G. Kaplan, J.B. Miller, I.P. Stiver, & J.L. Surrey (Eds.), *Women's growth in connection* (pp. 237–249). New York: The Guilford Press.

Surrey, J.L. (1991b). Relationship and empowerment. In J.V. Jordan, A.G. Kaplan, J.B. Miller, I.P. Stiver, & J.L. Surrey (Eds.), *Women's growth in connection* (pp. 162–180). New York: The Guilford Press.

Surrey, J.L. (1991c). The "self-in-relation": A theory of women's development. In J.V. Jordan, A.G. Kaplan, J.B. Miller, I.P. Stiver, & J.L. Surrey (Eds.), *Women's growth in connection* (pp. 51–66). New York: The Guilford Press.

Surrey, J.L. (1997). What do you mean by mutuality? In J.V. Jordan (Ed.), *Women's growth in diversity: More writings from the Stone Center* (pp. 42–49). New York: The Guilford Press.

Surrey, J.L., Kaplan, A., & Jordan, J.V. (1990). *Empathy revisited*. Wellesley, MA: The Stone Center.

Tantillo, M., Bitter, C.N., & Adams, B. (2001). Enhancing readiness for eating disorder treatment: A relational/motivational group model for change. *Eating Disorders*, 9, 203–216.

Tosone, C. (2013). On being a relational practitioner in an evidence-based world. *Journal of Social Work Practice*, 27(3), 249–257.

Tracy, E.M., Munson, M.R., Peterson, L.T., & Floersch, J.E. (2010). Social support: A mixed blessing for women in substance abuse treatment. *Journal of Social Work Practice in the Addictions*, 10(3), 257–282.

Tronick, E.Z. & Weinberg, M.K. (1997). Depressed mothers and infants: Failure to form dyadic states of consciousness. In L. Murray & P.J. Cooper (Eds.), *Postpartum depression and child development* (pp. 54–81). New York: The Guilford Press.

Tronto, J.C. (1993). An ethic of care. *Generations*, 22(3), 15–21.

Tropp, E. (1977). Social group work: The development approach. In J.B. Turner (Ed.), *Encyclopedia of social work, Vol. 11* (pp. 1321–1327). 17th Edition. Washington, DC: National Association of Social Workers.

Truax, C.B. & Mitchell, K.M. (1971). Research on certain therapist interpersonal skills in relation to process and outcome. In A.E. Bergin & S.L. Garfield (Eds.), *Handbook of psychotherapy and behavior change* (pp. 299–344). New York: John Wiley & Sons.

Turner, F. (2002). *Diagnosis in social work*. Binghamton, NY: Haworth Press.

Turner, J.B. (Ed.). (1977). *Encyclopedia of social work, Vol. 1*. 17th Edition. Washington, DC: National Association of Social Workers.

Walker, M. (2004). How relationships heal. In M. Walker & W.B. Rosen (Eds.), *How connections heal: Stories from relational–cultural therapy*, (pp. 3–22). New York: The Guilford Press.

Watson-Phillips, C. (2006). Relational fathering: How fathering sons affects men's relational growth and development. Poster session presented at the Jean Baker Miller Training Institute, Wellesley Centers for Women, Wellesley, MA.

Wenocur, S. & Reisch, M. (1989). *From charity to enterprise: The development of American social work in a market economy*. Urbana, IL: University of Illinois Press.

Werner, E.E. (1989). High-risk children in young adulthood: a longitudinal study from birth to 32 years. *American Journal of Orthopsychiatry*, 59(1), 72–81.

White, R. (1963). *Ego and reality in psychoanalytic theory*. New York: International Universities Press.

Winnicott, D.W. (1965). *The maturational processes and the facilitating environment*. New York: International Universities Press.

Wishnie, H.A. (2005). *Working in the counter-transference: Necessary entanglements*. Lanham, MD: Rowman & Littlefield.

Woods, M.E. & Hollis, F. (1999). *Casework: A psychosocial therapy*. 5th Edition. New York: McGraw-Hill.

Index

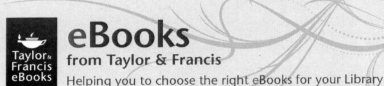
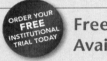
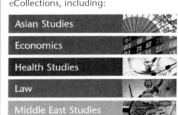

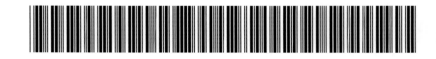

DATE DUE	RETURNED